Management of Headache and Headache Medications

Lawrence D. Robbins, M.D.

Management of Headache
and
Headache Medications

Foreword by Jerome Goldstein, M.D.

Springer—Verlag

New York Berlin Heidelberg London Paris
Tokyo Hong Kong Barcelona Budapest

Lawrence D. Robbins, M.D.
Assistant Professor of Neurology
Rush Medical College
Clinical Assistant Professor of Neurology
University of Illinois
Chicago, IL, USA
Director
Robbins Headache Clinic
Northbrook, IL, USA

Library of Congress Cataloging-in-Publication Data
Robbins, Lawrence D.
    Management of headache and headache medications / Lawrence D.
Robbins.
        p.   cm.
    Includes bibliographical references and index.
    ISBN 0-387-94040-5. — ISBN 3-540-94040-5
    1. Headache—Chemotherapy.   I. Title.
    [DNLM: 1. Headache—drug therapy.   2. Headache—prevention &
control.   WL 342 R634m 1993]
    RB128.R63   1993
    616.8'491—dc20
    DNLM/DLC
    for Library of Congress   93-19226

Printed on acid-free paper.

Production managed by Dimitry L. Loseff; Manufacturing supervised by Vincent Scelta.
Typeset by Best-set Typesetter Ltd., Hong Kong.
Printed and bound by Edwards Brothers, Ann Arbor, MI.
Printed in the United States of America.

9 8 7 6 5 4 3 2 1

ISBN 0-387-94040-5 Springer-Verlag New York Berlin Heidelberg
ISBN 3-540-94040-5 Springer-Verlag Berlin Heidelberg New York

Dedicated to Headache Sufferers
and Their Families

Thanks to Sharon, Mom, and Dad

Foreword

The art of treating headache patients is a complex one, and there are a myriad of medication possibilities. Dr. Robbins has managed to present a clear and practical approach to headache medicines. He brings us through standard first line therapies into more complex "end of the line" medication treatments.

This book presents a cohesive, single-authored approach that is unique. Illustrative case histories and "Quick Reference Guides" are extremely useful, and Dr. Robbins has inserted thousands of practical tips on headache management, advice that is impossible to find in other sources.

Preventive and abortive medication for migraine, tension, and cluster headache are completely discussed. Hormonal aspects, such as treatment of menstrual and menopausal headache, are presented at length. There is an extensive section on children's headaches, and a separate discussion on headache in adolescents. These sections present a very clear and effective approach to headache management in children and adolescents. Dr. Robbins effectively tackles such important subjects as post-traumatic headache, lumbar puncture headache, indomethacin responsive syndromes, and occipital neuralgia.

Dr. Lawrence Robbins is one of our top authorities on the management of headache medications. He has contributed greatly through his research and writing on various headache topics. This book will be invaluable for those involved in the treatment of patients with headache.

Jerome Goldstein, M.D.
Assistant Clinical Professor of Neurology,
University of California, San Francisco.
Director, San Francisco Headache Clinic,
San Francisco.

Preface

There exists a confusing array of headache medications. Each headache sufferer is unique and requires a different medication regimen. There is a delicate art to managing these medications. This book presents a logical approach to successfully managing headache patients.

We need to view headache as a medical condition that may be affected by stress or psychological factors. Treating headache as a psychological condition has been unsuccessful and generally drives patients to seek help elsewhere. The patients do need to be educated about their condition, and taught nonmedical approaches such as diet and relaxation. I discuss these measures in Chapter 1. For most headache patients, the success or failure of treatment lies in the efficacy of the medication regimen.

The majority of this book describes treatment for migraine, chronic daily (tension), and cluster headache. I have included extensive sections on hormonal aspects of headache, headache in children and adolescents, and "special" headache situations, such as headache in the elderly. Case histories are presented, along with "Quick Reference Guides" prior to major sections.

For the physician, treating headache patients primarily involves changing and managing a complicated array of medications, being willing to switch medicines, and having the patience to stick with the headache sufferer. Our goal is to improve the quality of life for those afflicted with headache. This goal can be accomplished in almost all headache patients.

Lawrence Robbins, M.D.

Contents

CHAPTER 1

Introduction to Migraine

Definition and Characteristics of Migraine

Migraine with aura and migraine without aura have replaced the older terms "classical migraine" and "nonclassical migraine." In my treatment of migraine, I usually do not differentiate between migraine with or without aura, as the therapy generally remains the same. Migraine without aura is a chronic idiopathic headache disorder with attacks lasting 4 to 72 hours. Status migrainosis applies to migraine headaches that exceed 72 hours in length. Migraine features often include unilateral location; moderate, moderate-to-severe, or severe intensity of the pain; and a throbbing or pulsating nature to the pain. There may be associated nausea, photophobia, or phonophobia. Migraine in first-degree relatives (70% to 75% of migraine patients report a first-degree relative having had migraine), positive relationship with menses, decreased frequency during pregnancy, and increase of the pain with physical activity are further characteristics. (See Table 1.1)

A recurring headache that is moderate or severe and is triggered by migraine precipitating factors is usually considered to be migraine. These factors include stress, certain foods, weather changes, smoke, hunger, fatigue, etc. Migraineurs often have colder hands and feet than controls, and the prevalence of motion sickness is much higher in migraine patients. Patients usually do not have all of the above characteristics, and there are certain diagnostic criteria that have been established by the International Headache Society for the definite diagnosis of migraine. Many patients do not have nausea, photophobia, or phonophobia. Distinguishing a milder migraine without aura from a moderate or severe tension headache may be very difficult, and I am not surprised when "pure" migraine medications are effective for severe tension headaches. I generally regard recurrent, repeated attacks of throbbing or severe aching headache as migraine, whether or not the patient has nausea, photophobia, or phono-phobia. We are assuming that organic disorders, particularly brain tumors, have been ruled out or excluded. Twenty percent of women and 7% of men experience recurring migraine headaches at some point during their lifetime. The peak ages are between 20 and 35 years old.

TABLE 1.1. Characteristics of Migraine.

Attacks are 4 to 72 hours
Moderate or moderate-to-severe pain
History by the patient gives the diagnosis, not lab tests
Often early morning, but may be anytime
Unilateral in one half of patients
One to five migraines per month is typical
Gradual onset of pain, a peak for hours, slow decline
Pain is throbbing, pounding, pulsatile, or deep aching
Sharp "ice-pick" jabs are common
Peak ages are between 20 and 35 years
20% of women, 7% of men experience migraine in their lifetime; female/male ratio is 3:1
Family history is often positive for migraine
Associated nausea, photophobia, blurred vision, phonophobia, dizziness is common; however, these may be absent
In women, there is often a positive relationship with menses, and decreased headaches during pregnancy
Cold hands and feet, or motion sickness is common in migraine patients

The patient's history gives us the diagnosis of migraine. Physical exam and MRI or CAT scans are helpful only in ruling out organic pathology. Although migraine headaches may begin at any time during the day, they often begin early in the morning, upon awakening. Headaches that awaken patients and are of recent onset need to be investigated with an MRI scan. A check of intraocular pressure may be warranted. Although the pain is unilateral in 50% of migraineurs, the entire head often becomes involved. The pain may be in the facial or cervical areas, and often will shift sides from one occurrence to another. Most patients, however, suffer the severe pain on one favored side from attack to attack.

The typical migraine patient suffers one to five attacks per month, but many patients average less than one or more than 10 per month. The attack frequency varies with the seasons, and many patients can identify the time of year when their headaches increase significantly.

The pain of the migraine often follows a bell shaped curve, with a gradual ascent, a peak for a number of hours (or longer), and then a slow decline. Occasionally the pain may be at its peak within minutes of the onset.

Migraine pain is often throbbing, pounding, or pulsatile, particularly when the patient's head is bent. The pain may simply be a steady, severe ache. Jabs of sharp pain, lasting seconds, are frequently experienced by migraineurs.

Most patients with migraine suffer some degree of nausea during the attack, and many patients have vomiting as well. The nausea is often mild, and some migraineurs are not bothered by it. Many patients state that the headache is lessened after they vomit. Diarrhea occurs in some

TABLE 1.2. Somatic Symptoms Accompanying Migraine.

Listed in order of frequency
  Sensitivity to light
  Blurred vision
  Nausea
  Tenderness about the scalp
  Dizziness or lightheadedness
  Lethargy
  Vomiting
  Retention of fluid, with weight gain
  Photopsia
  Vertigo
  Anxiety
  Paresthesias
  Diarrhea
  Fortification spectra
  Nasal stuffiness
  Mild aphasia
  Syncope or near syncope
  Severe confusion
  Seizures
  Fever
  Hemiparesis or hemiplegia
  Ataxia and/or dysarthria (brain stem dysfunction)

patients, and is usually mild to moderate. The presence of diarrhea renders the use of rectal suppositories very difficult. (See Table 1.2)

Lightheadedness often accompanies the migraine, and syncope may occur; some patients pass out regularly with their attacks. Most patients become very sensitive to bright lights, sounds, and to odors. In between migraine attacks, many patients retain the photophobia, and it is common for migraine patients to wear sunglasses most of the time. Sensitivity to bright lights is a distinctive migraine characteristic.

Pallor of the face is common during a migraine; flushing may occur as well, but is seen less often. Patients often complain of feeling excessively hot or cold during an attack, and the skin temperature may increase or decrease on the side of the pain. Migraineurs often have cold hands and/or feet at all times.

Migraineurs often experience tenderness of the scalp that may linger on for hours or days after the migraine pain has ceased. This tenderness may actually occur during the prodrome of the migraine. Both vascular and muscular factors contribute to the scalp tenderness.

Mild elevations in temperature are more commonly seen with migraines than is generally appreciated. Autonomic disturbances are relatively common, such as pupillary miosis or dilatation, rhinorrhea, eye tearing, and nasal stuffiness. These are also symptoms of cluster headache, and migraineurs often experience aspects of cluster headache, including the sharp pain about one eye or temple.

Alterations in mood are seen with many patients prior to, during, and after migraine attacks. Patients are usually anxious, tired, or depressed. They often feel "washed out" after an attack, but a calm or euphoric state occasionally is seen as a postdrome to the migraine. Rarely, euphoria or exhilaration may precede a migraine.

Weight gain due to fluid retention is common, and begins prior to the migraine. At some point during the migraine, patients often experience polyuria. The weight gain is usually less than 6 pounds, and is transient.

Visual Disturbances

Blurred vision is very common during migraine attacks, and is usually only mild or moderate. Approximately 40% of patients experience visual neurologic disturbances preceding or during the migraine; these auras may be as disturbing to the patient as the migraine pain itself. Most migraineurs experience the same aura with each migraine, but occasionally one person may have several types of auras. "The light of a flash bulb going off" is the description that many migraineurs give to their aura. The visual hallucinations seen most often consist of spots, stars, lines (often wavy), color splashes, and waves resembling heat waves. The images may seem to shimmer, sparkle, or flicker. The above visual occurences are referred to as photopsia.

Fortification spectra are seen much less often than photopsia. They usually begin with a decrease in vision and visual hallucinations that are unformed. Within minutes, a paracentral scotoma becomes evident, and this assumes a crescent shape, usually with "zig-zags." There is often associated shimmering, sparkling, or flickering at the edges of the scotoma.

Patients may experience a "graying out" of their vision, or a "whiteout" may occur. Some patients suffer complete visual loss, usually for some minutes. Photopsia may be experienced at the same time as the gray out, whiteout, or visual loss.

The visual symptoms usually last 15 to 20 minutes, and most often will be followed by the migraine headache. Visual symptoms without the headache are common, and are often very distressing to the patient.

Miscellaneous Neurologic Symptoms Associated with Migraine

Numbness or tingling (paresthesias) are commonnly experienced as part of the migraine. These are most often experienced in one hand and forearm, but may be felt in the face, periorally, or in both arms and legs. Like the visual disturbances, they often last only minutes preceeding the pain, but the numbness may go on for hours, and at times the paresthesias are severe. The sensory disturbances usually increase slowly over 15 to

25 minutes, differentiating them from the more rapid pace seen with epilepsy.

Paralysis of the limbs may occur, but this is rare. This is occasionally seen as a familial autosomal dominant trait, and the term familial hemiplegic migraine is applied to this form. With the weakness, aphasia or slurred speech may also occur, and sensory disturbances are seen ipsilateral to the weakness.

Vertigo is occasionally experienced during the attack of migraine, and may be disabling. Ataxia may occur, but is not common. Rarely, multiple symptoms of brain stem dysfunction may occur, with the term basilar migraine being applied to this type of syndrome. The attack usually begins with visual disturbances (most often photopsia), followed by ataxia, vertigo, paresthesias, and other brain stem symptoms. After 15 to 30 minutes, these severe neurologic symptoms usually abate, and are followed by a headache. This type of migraine often stops over months or years, and the patient is simply left with migraine headaches without neurologic dysfunction.

Workup for Migraine

When patients present with a long history of typical migraine attacks, and the headaches are essentially unchanged, scans of the head are usually not absolutely necessary. The issue of testing for migraine has presented legal problems, for chronic migraine patients may develop a brain tumor that is unrelated to the headache, and the legal system in the United States is very poor at deciding whether the physician was at fault for not obtaining a test. The preferred head scan for migraine is a MRI. The current ability to noninvasively obtain an angiogram (MRA) with the MRI allows us to detect most intracranial aneurysms.

Situations that raise the concern about organic pathology (see Table 1.3) include: (1) progressive headaches over days or weeks, increasing in intensity; (2) new onset headaches, particularly in patients who "never" have headaches, or new onset exertional headaches; (3) neurologic symptoms or signs, stiff neck, papilledema, and changes in level of consciousness; (4) fever that is not explained; (5) radical increase or change in a preexisting headache pattern.

TABLE 1.3. Situations that Raise the Concern About Organic Pathology.

1. Progressive headaches over days or weeks, increasing in intensity
2. New onset headaches, particularly in patients who never have headaches
3. New onset headaches with exertion
4. Neurologic symptoms or signs, stiff neck, papilledema, and changes in level of consciousness
5. Fever that is not explained
6. Radical increase or change in a preexisting headache pattern

TABLE 1.4. Factors That May Trigger Migraine.

Stress, worry, or acute anxiety
Hormonal factors, such as menstruation, birth control pill, pregnancy, menopause, estrogens
Weather changes
Diet
Fatigue or lack of sleep
Missing a meal
Smoke, perfumes, gasoline, paint, or organic solvents
Oversleeping
Exertion, exercise, or sex
Bright lights
Trauma to the head

The tests that are generally useful for diagnosis of headache are the MRI (brain) scan, the CAT (brain) scan, lumbar puncture, intraocular pressure testing, radiography or CAT scans of the sinuses, and blood tests. MRA is becoming very valuable in the diagnosis of aneurysms. Whether to do any testing at all depends upon the physician's clinical suspicion of organic pathology. Although some patients request a "test" of their head, the vast majority of chronic migraineurs state that "if I had a brain tumor I would be dead years ago." Sound clinical judgement, based on patient history and a physical exam, is crucial in deciding who needs which exam.

The problems that need to be excluded in a patient with a "new onset" of migraine include: sinus disease, meningitis, glaucoma, brain tumor, arteritis, subarachnoid hemorrhage, idiopathic intracranial hypertension, hydrocephalus, pheochromocytoma, stroke or TIA, internal carotid artery dissection, and systemic illnesses. Excluding most of these problems is usually easily accomplished by the history and physical exam.

Factors That May Trigger Migraine

The trigger factors for migraine are many and varied. (See Table 1.4) They will not consistently trigger migraines, but the factors are additive; i.e., if there is a weather change and a severe stress has occurred. A food, for instance, might trigger a migraine one month and not the next. Some patients are not able to identify more than one trigger factor, and others have multiple precipitating factors. The more common migraine triggers will be discussed. It should be recognized that the vast majority of migraines are not associated with any easily identifiable precipitating factor.

Stress, Worry, and Anxiety

In patients who do have the physical illness that we consider migraine, a severe stress may precipitate a migraine. A new anxiety provoking situation will often bring on a headache. Many patients suffer the migraine after the stress is over, which is termed a "let-down" headache. Weekend headaches are common in migraineurs who work Monday through Friday. Migraine patients are much more likely than controls to develop anxiety-panic disorder, which probably underscores the crucial role of serotonin in both disorders. Although emotional factors may exacerbate illness, it is clear that migraine is an inherited, physical illness. Patients who are experiencing severe, recurring head pain may become secondarily depressed about the situation. Depression in headache patients is not usually the cause of their pain, but may render the patients more likely to have an increased frequency of headache.

Until emotional stresses are resolved, it is likely that the headaches will continue to be exacerbated. Workplace or home conflicts are constant triggers for the headache.

Psychotherapy may help headache patients in a variety of ways: the patient may learn to cope more effectively, to deal with stresses appropriately, to resolve interpersonal conflicts, to modify perfectionistic behavior, and learn to deal with anger and other repressed emotions. However, therapy may not directly decrease the headaches, and patients are often frustrated when they are told that psychotherapy may improve the pain.

Many patients do not have the willingness or insight to proceed with psychotherapy. Patients often cite time and money as reasons not to see a therapist or to learn relaxation techniques. Group therapy is less expensive and, at times, more productive than individual counseling. Although many patients could benefit from psychotherapy, relatively few are actually willing to put the time, effort, and money into therapy.

Relaxation Techniques and Headache

Relaxation and/or biofeedback techniques are usually helpful for those patients who are willing to do the deep breathing, imagery, or muscle relaxation exercises. Simple relaxation training, primarily utilizing deep breathing, is easy to learn, and most patients can effectively learn this at home. There is little need for multisession, expensive biofeedback training programs, because experience and studies have shown us that a simple home-based program is just as effective. In general, the younger the patient, the more successful relaxation therapy will be, but the success of relaxation is directly tied to the motivation of the person. Patients should certainly be encouraged to try deep breathing, if only for 10 or 20 seconds, instead of automatically reaching for a pill.

A major problem with existing biofeedback programs is the time and money involved. When we suggest a formal biofeedback training program for patients, only a tiny fraction of people actually follow through. However, when patients receive a simple booklet describing breathing, im-

TABLE 1.5. Relaxation Therapy for Headache.

Useful for headache, neck pain, nervousness, stress, tension
Deep breathing and imagery are most important
Patients should be encouraged to do 20 or 30 seconds of relaxation when they feel tension or
  headache building
Booklets and cassette tapes need to be made available to patients for a home-based
  program; they will not usually undertake an expensive biofeedback program
Children and adolescents should particularly be encouraged to learn relaxation/biofeedback

aging, and muscle relaxation techniques, many more patients are willing
to at least attempt to utilize the exercises. One or two sessions with a
psychotherapist who is able to teach relaxation may help to a great
extent. The therapist will often produce a relaxation cassette for the
patient. If patients are willing to do the deep breathing, if only for
seconds, and utilize the relaxation techniques on a regular basis, they
often achieve some benefit from the exercises. The trick is to make these

TABLE 1.6. Foods That Are Common Migraine Triggers.

Monosodium Glutamate (MSG): also labeled Autolyzed Yeast Extract, Hydrolyzed
  Vegetable Protein, or Natural Flavoring. Possible sources of MSG include: broths or
  stock, seasonings, whey protein, soy extract, malt extract, caseinate, barley extract,
  textured soy protein, chicken, pork, or beef flavoring, smoke flavor, spices, carrageenan,
  meat tenderizer, seasoned salt, TV dinners, instant gravies, and some potato chips and
  dry-roasted nuts.
Red wine
Chocolate
Citrus fruits
Ripened, aged cheeses (cheddar, bleu, brick, Colby, Roquefort, brie, Gruyere, mozzarella,
  Parmesan, boursalt, Romano). Cottage cheese, cream cheese, and American cheese are
  much less likely to trigger headache.
Processed cheese
Hot dogs, pepperoni, bologna, salami, sausage, canned or aged meats, cured meats (bacon,
  ham), marinated meats
White wine
Beer
Alcohol (miscellaneous); vodka is the least likely to bring on migraine
Cocoa
Fresh, hot, homemade yeast breads (once cooled they are OK)
Buttermilk
Chocolate milk
Sour cream
Yogurt
Caffeine (usually, caffeine helps headaches; too much caffeine causes increased, rebound
  headaches. Some migraineurs are extremely sensitive to small amounts of caffeine.)
Yeast extracts
Acidophilus milk

techniques easily accessible and affordable. In occasional circumstances, such as with certain children, extended sessions of biofeedback training are the only manner in which the person will effectively learn the techniques. Relaxation techniques are provided in the Appendix.

Diet

In many migraineurs, dietary trigger factors will occasionally bring on a headache. The degree of sensitivity to foods varies widely among migraine sufferers. The mechanism of food-provoked headaches is probably not an allergy, but rather a sensitivity to chemicals in the foods, such as tyramine, phenylethylamine (in chocolate), and monosodium glutamate. Nitrites may also be a problem.

The headache will usually begin soon after ingestion of the offending substance, but there may be a delay of hours. At certain times, patients may be more susceptible to the foods, such as a female migraineur around menstruation. Trigger factors are usually "additive" for migraine. Patients should be made aware of the foods that might be trigger factors and instructed to avoid them for a period of time, and then to add them back, noting the ones that trigger their migraines. Foods should not be over-emphasized, as it is easy for migraineurs to become obsessed with watching their diet. Patients are often then frustrated and disappointed, because they state that "I watched all of the foods like a hawk, and I still have headaches. I don't understand." Migraineurs need to be made aware that the foods are but one of many influencing factors on migraine.

Tables 1.6 and 1.7 list foods that, at times, may trigger headaches.

TABLE 1.7. Foods that Trigger Migraine Less Often.

Onions
Certain beans: lima, navy, fava, lentils, garbanzo, pinto, Italian, and snow peas
Sauerkraut
Pickles
Chile peppers
Licorice or carob candy
Figs, raisins, avocado, banana, passion fruit, papaya
Liver
Fried foods
Peanuts, peanut butter
Popcorn
Nuts or seeds
Soy sauce
Sugar in excess
Salt in excess
Seafood
Pork
Aspartame

Weather Changes

Spring tends to be the worst season for migraine sufferers, followed by fall. The hot, humid days of summer also may precipitate migraines. Many patients state that when the weather changes they often experience a migraine. The severity of migraines may be more influenced by weather than the frequency of the headaches. Although there have been conflicting studies on weather and headache, the weight of evidence favors weather being a major precipitating factor in migraine; however, most migraine headaches are not precipitated by any identifiable occurrence.

Fatigue or Lack of Sleep

This factor is particularly important in children as a migraine precipitant. When migraineurs are awakened early in the morning, particularly by a bright light, they often will experience a migraine. It is very helpful if the headache patient is able to achieve consistent sleep; when people change time shifts on their job, they often experience migraines during the adjustment period.

Missing a Meal

Most migraineurs realize that if they do miss meals they are more likely to encounter some type of headache as a result. It is very important for migraine prone people to eat regularly, usually at least 3 times per day.

Hormonal Factors

Hormonal factors, including birth control pills, pregnancy, menopause, estrogens, and, particularly, menstruation, often play a crucial role in precipitating migraines in women. The headaches are usually improved during pregnancy. Menstruation-related migraines are often the most severe, and tend to be difficult to effectively treat.

This subject is covered extensively in Chapter 4.

Smoke, Perfumes, Gasoline, and Paint Organic Solvents

These may trigger tension or migraine headaches in susceptible individuals. The sensitivity to cigarette smoke may develop at anytime in one's life, even in people who previously were smokers. Many people cannot tolerate exposure to even small amounts of perfumes or gasoline. The magazines that contain perfumes in the pages are often a hazard for migraine prone patients. Paint smells are common triggers for migraine.

Oversleeping

In adults, excessive sleep may lead to a migraine attack. This factor does not seem to be important in children and adolescents. Although sleep will often stop a migraine, too much sleep is a problem. Regulating sleep is important, particularly on weekends. Naps may be a problem with some patients. As much as one half hour of extra sleep on a Sunday morning may be enough to trigger a migraine after a stressful week.

Exertion, Exercise, and Sex

In some patients, certain types of exertion may consistently trigger migraines. The headache usually occurs within minutes of finishing the exercise. Sexual headaches are common. Anti-inflammatories taken prior to the exercise or sex often prevent the headache. Exertional and sexual headaches are discussed at length in Chapter 13.

Bright Lights

Most migraine patients are sensitive to bright flourescent light and sunlight, even when they do not have a migraine. Migraineurs wear sunglasses much more often than nonheadache prone individuals. The glare of the sun while driving may trigger a migraine. Camera flashes are common precipitants of auras or migraine headaches. At times, migraineurs have trouble with the bright flouresent lights of grocery stores. The glare of a computer is a problem for some people if they need to sit in front of the screen for extended periods.

Trauma to the Head

A blow to the head may trigger migraines in both migraineurs and people with no history of headache. Rear end whiplash accidents are a common source of headache that may be present for months or years. Post-traumatic headache is covered extensively in Chapter 13.

Pathogenesis of Migraine

Migraine pathophysiology is unknown at this point. We have several concepts that have emerged over the years that can be divided into two categories: the vascular versus the neural theories. Unfortunately, only 5% (or less) of what needs to be known scientifically has actually been discovered; in 10 years, we will have changed our perception of migraine events in the body, and in 20 years that perception will be outdated. The following will briefly review several of the known concepts.

Vascular Concept of Migraine

For many years, migraines were attributed to vasospasm, followed by inflammation and vasodilation. Vasodilation of the larger arteries and veins was thought to be due in part to arteriovenous shunting. The initial vasospasm was long held to be responsible for the migraine aura. Extracranial vessel dilatation is undoubtedly a factor in the pain of migraine, but to what extent is not known.

Hypoperfusion of the cerebral cortex does occur in classic migraine, and this lasts for hours. The hypoperfusion is mild to moderate, and slowly spreads along the cortical convolutions. It is not known how often ischemic levels are reached. It is most likely that the blood flow changes that are observed are a result, not a cause, of primary neuronal factors.

Role of the Trigeminal Nerve

Vessel innervation about the cranium is primarily derived from the ipsilateral trigeminal nerve. Substance P is released by the trigeminovascular fibers when they are stimulated. This triggers the inflammatory response. Other neurotransmitters are involved in the trigeminovascular system, including somatostatin and cholecystokinin.

This trigeminovascular system is involved in generating a portion of the pain of migraine. The primary neuronal events that trigger this system to respond can only be speculated upon.

Serotonin

During migraine, urinary serotonin levels increase and platelet serotonin levels diminish. In the cerebral vasculature, serotonin is a vasoconstrictor. Small arteries and large arterioles in the cerebral circulation are constricted by serotonin; small pial arterioles dilate. Most of the serotonergic cells lie within the midline of the brain stem. From this small area, projections terminate to most portions of the cerebrum. When these midline (raphe) nuclei are stimulated, there is a decrease in the rate of firing of cerebral neurons. Serotonin is usually inhibitory and a number of different serotonin receptors have been identified. Certain antimigraine drugs bind to serotonin receptors. It is possible that a major aspect of migraine involves dysfunction in the modulating system of serotonin in the brainstem raphe area. The increased activity of the serotonergic raphe cells may then lead to the circulatory changes typically seen in migraine.

The pathophysiology of migraine will be delineated more clearly in the next 50 years. Since the basis for the pain remains somewhat unclear, the mechanism of action of antimigraine drugs can only be speculated upon. In this book, I do not delve into mechanisms of action, because to do this with our current base of knowledge is probably not accurate for the majority of our migraine medicines.

CHAPTER 2

Migraine Abortive Medication

Sleep, a dark and quiet room, and reusable ice packs applied to the pain are very helpful for migraine headache. Caffeine, such as in coffee or caffeine tablets, may also lessen the pain. Most patients require an abortive medication. A bewildering variety of medication choices are available for aborting migraine headaches. For a number of patients, simple preparations consisting of aspirin or ibuprofen are all that are needed. The goal is to decrease pain and nausea while producing a minimum of side effects. In migraine, the earlier a medication is taken, the more effective it is. The nausea of the migraine may preclude the use of aspirin or anti-inflammatory compounds, but in general these compounds are more effective than acetaminophen.

The serotonin agonists dihydroergotamine (DHE) and sumatriptan are the most effective migraine abortives. The older ergotamines, such as Cafergot, are also very helpful. However, because of ease of administration and favorable side effect profiles, the following are the first line abortive medications: (1) NSAIDs, (2) Midrin, (3) aspirin plus caffeine compounds, (4) butalbital medications.

The choice as to which first line abortive to use, or whether to jump to a second line abortive, depends upon many factors. These include the age of the patient (we avoid the ergotamines, except DHE and sumatriptan, after age 40 or so), nausea (with nausea being prominent, aspirin or NSAIDs are best avoided; Midrin, Esgic, or DHE are better choices), and, if the patient needs to continue working and functioning, nonsedating medications are preferred.

In certain situations, we can formulate specific preparations that are not commercially available. If patients are not able to swallow a pill, a compounding pharmacist is able to make an oral lozenge or a rectal suppository that will deliver any medication combination that we need. By utilizing the compounding pharmacists, we are not limited to commercially available medications for migraine.

Most of the medications widely used for migraine have not received specific FDA indications for this use. The following is only a guide to

TABLE 2.1. Quick Reference Guide: First Line Migraine Abortive Medication.

1. Excedrin (Extra Strength): useful as an over-the-counter preparation with aspirin, caffeine, and acetaminophen. Anxiety from the caffeine, or nausea from the aspirin is common. One or two pills every 3 hours as needed is effective for many patients with mild or moderate migraines. Aspirin Free Excedrin is also available, but is less effective. This contains acetaminophen plus caffeine.
2. Naproxen (Anaprox [DS]): Useful in younger patients, occasionally helpful for menstrual migraine. Nonsedating, but very frequent GI upset. The usual dose is Anaprox DS (550 mg), one tablet with food or Tums to start, then may repeat in 1 hour (if no severe nausea), and then in 3 or 4 hours. Three per day at most.
3. Ibuprofen: Over the counter, and approved for children. Liquid Advil is available. Not as effective as Anaprox. Occasionally useful in menstrual migraine. GI side effects are common. The usual dose is 400 to 800 mg every 3 hours, limiting the total dose to 2,400 mg per day. Combining with caffeine may be helpful.
4. Midrin: Effective, safe, and used in children. Fatigue is common. Contains a vasoconstrictor, a nonaddicting sedative, and acetaminophen. Usual dose is one or two pills to start, then one every hour as needed, five or six per day at most. May be combined with caffeine for increased efficacy. Generally well tolerated.
5. Norgesic Forte: Effective nonaddicting combination of aspirin, caffeine, and orphenadrine. GI side effects are common, as is fatigue. Usual dose is one-half or one tablet every 3 or 4 hours, four per day at most.
6. Fiorinal, Fioricet, Esgic: Fiorinal contains ASA, butalbital, and caffeine; Fioricet and Esgic replace the ASA with acetaminophen. Generics of these compounds do not work well. These are addicting, but very effective for many patients. Dosage is one or two pills every 3 hours, with a limit of 30 or 40 pills per month at most. Fiorinal with codeine (#3) adds 30 mg of codeine, and is more effective than plain Fiorinal.

what I consider reasonable and rational therapy for headache. Prior to prescribing medications for patients, they need to be informed of, and accept, the complete set of contraindications and side effects as listed in the PDR and package insert.

First Line Abortive Medication

Extra Strength (E.S.) Excedrin

Although it is a very effective over the counter (OTC) preparation of acetaminophen (250 mg), aspirin (250 mg), and caffeine (65 mg), Excedrin E.S. should not be over-used on a daily basis, as it may create rebound headaches. Nephrotoxicity or hepatic irritation is also a concern. If Excedrin is used every day, the limit should be an average of two pills per day. If patients require more than this, consideration should be given to daily prevention medication. The combination of acetaminophen, aspirin, and caffeine increases the potential for renal problems with chronic abuse. Excedrin E.S. contains more caffeine than does Anacin, rendering it more effective, but this can also lead to caffeine rebound headaches.

Dosage

One or two tablets every 3 hours as needed.

Side Effects

Nausea, stomach pain, heartburn, or anxiety are common. Long term daily use may predispose to renal problems or gastric bleeding.

Aspirin Free Excedrin

A combination of acetaminophen (250 mg) plus caffeine (65 mg), Aspirin Free Excedrin eliminates the GI side effects of aspirin. Although not as effective as Excedrin E.S., for patients with ulcers or excessive nausea this is a useful product. Dosage is usually two pills every 3 to 4 hours. This very well tolerated medication seldom produces side effects other than the anxiety or insomnia from caffeine.

Naproxen Sodium (Anaprox)

Each tablet of Anaprox Double Strength (DS) contains 550 mg of naproxen, a very effective drug for various types of headache. It is particularly helpful around the menstrual period, and with caution may be used for daily headaches as well. Naproxen is also employed as a daily preventive medication. Adding caffeine, either coffee or one pill of a 100 mg caffeine tablet (No-Doz), may add to the effectiveness of naproxen.

Dosage

One pill to start, then one more pill may be taken in 1 hour if needed, and then 3 or 4 hours after the second, three per day at most. If the Anaprox is well tolerated, as many as two pills may be taken at the onset, with another (if needed) in 3 or 4 hours. Pills should be taken with something to eat, or with an antacid or Tums. When used as a preventive, the dosage is usually one or two pills per day.

Side Effects

Nausea and GI upset are common. Metoclopramide (Reglan), 5 or 10 mg, or promethazine (Phenergan), 25 mg, taken prior to or with the Anaprox may relieve the nausea. Serious side effects (GI, liver, renal) may occur when naproxen is taken on a daily basis for extended periods of time. It is useful in younger patients, but serious side effects are more common in older age groups.

Ibuprofen (Motrin)

This anti-inflammatory is occasionally helpful and is reasonably well tolerated. Ibuprofen is available over the counter. Dosage varies from 200 to 800 mg every 3 hours. Side effects, such as the frequent GI upset, are very similar to naproxen. The relatively low cost and OTC availability render ibuprofen helpful for some patients. Adding caffeine may enhance the effectiveness of ibuprofen.

Ketorolac Pills (Toradol)

Early experience with this relatively new anti-inflammatory has indicated that ketorolac is helpful for certain patients when other anti-inflammatories have not been effective. One or two pills are taken with food at the onset, and then one every 3 hours up to a maximum of four per day. Ketorolac should not be used on a daily basis. The number of ketorolac pills needs to be limited per month because of the potential for hepatic or renal toxicity. Ketorolac needs to be discontinued if abdominal pain occurs, and it should not be used in patients with hepatic or renal impairment.

Midrin

An extremely effective, well tolerated medication, Midrin consists of a vasoconstrictor, isometheptane, combined with dichloralphenazone, a nonaddicting sedative, and 250 mg of acetaminophen. It may be given to children over 5 years of age, as well as to the elderly. For most migraine patients, Midrin should be utilized early in their migraine course. Adding caffeine, either strong coffee or one-half to one pill of a 100 mg caffeine tablet (No-Doz) may help offset the fatigue often seen with Midrin. Caffeine also enhances the analgesic effect.

Dosage

One or two capsules at the onset of the headache, then one capsule is repeated every hour as needed up to a maximum of six per day and 20 per week. When using Midrin for the first time, patients should try one capsule first, because fatigue or lightheadedness may be overwhelming with two capsules. The capsules may be pulled apart, with one-half capsule used in applesauce or yogurt, or simply taken by itself. This is useful for children and in patients who have a difficult time swallowing the large Midrin capsule. The generic Midrin is not as effective as the regular Midrin; this seems to be true for many pain medications used for headache.

Side Effects

Fatigue or mild GI upset are common. Many patients complain of feeling lightheaded or "spacy." Midrin can raise the blood pressure, and must be used very cautiously in patients with hypertension. Midrin is generally well tolerated. It is the capsule that irritates the GI tract, and using only the Midrin powder inside may eliminate GI upset.

Norgesic Forte

Norgesic is an aspirin and caffeine combination with the addition of orphenadrine, a nonaddicting muscle relaxant. Norgesic Forte contains 770 mg of aspirin, 60 mg of caffeine, and 50 mg of orphenadrine. This is one of the more potent non-addicting abortive medications.

Dosage

One-half to one pill every 3 hours as needed, up to a maximum of four pills a day. Norgesic Forte pills are very large, and are scored. Because of the high aspirin content, Norgesic should be taken with food or an antacid. The Norgesic Forte brand is more effective than generic, which is generally true for the migraine abortives.

Side Effects

Nausea or fatigue may occur. Lightheadedness or "spaciness" are common. If nausea is a major accompaniment of the migraine, it is best to avoid Norgesic Forte as well as other aspirin-containing preparations. Abdominal pain may occur because of the high aspirin content. Blurred vision is occasionally seen, due to the orphenadrine.

Butalbital Compounds

Butalbital compounds are effective medications and include Fiorinal, Fioricet, Esgic, Esgic Plus, and Phrenilin. Fiorinal with codeine (Fiorinal #3) is also available. Addiction is a potential problem, but when used sparingly as needed for migraines, these medications are safe and often effective. Fiorinal, Esgic, and Phrenilin are variously formulated, and each has its own place in migraine therapy. In general, Fiorinal is more effective than Esgic, which is more effective than Phrenilin. However, each of these has specific uses, as is explained below. The generic butalbital compounds are best avoided, as they are not as effective as the brand name drugs in this class.

Fiorinal

Fiorinal contains 50 mg of butalbital, 325 mg of aspirin, and 40 mg of caffeine. The sedative effect of butalbital is usually offset by the caffeine.

Fiorinal is the most effective of the butalbital compounds, because aspirin is more effective than acetaminophen. Many patients experience a brief "high" or euphoria that can lead to addiction.

When patients begin to take the medication merely to relieve stress or anxiety, they need to discontinue use of butalbital compounds. Monthly limits need to be set for patients utilizing addicting compounds.

Dosage

Dosage is usually one or two pills every 3 hours as needed. I usually limit Fiorinal to 2 days per week; if patients do find it extremely useful for daily headaches, and other approaches have not been helpful, a monthly maximum needs to be explained to the patient. Forty pills per month is the usual maximum allotted, but this may be increased in unusual circumstances.

Side Effects

Fatigue, lightheadedness, "spaciness", and nausea are seen relatively often. Anxiety due to the caffeine may occur, but this effect is uncommon. Euphoria is common. The anxiety-reducing effect of Fiorinal and the butalbital compounds leads to occasional abuse. The aspirin may cause nausea or abdominal pain. Occasionally, patients who are not able to tolerate aspirin can tolerate Fiorinal, possibly because the butalbital may lessen the adverse GI effects of the aspirin.

Esgic, Fioricet, and Esgic Plus

Esgic and Fioricet have the same chemical composition: 50 mg of butalbital, 325 mg of acetaminophen, and 40 mg of caffeine. They are different from Fiorinal in that they contain acetaminophen instead of aspirin. Esgic Plus is the same as Esgic, with additional acetaminophen. The substitution of acetaminophen for aspirin renders Esgic and Fioricet less effective than Fiorinal, but also less troublesome as far as nausea is concerned. As mentioned, the generic butalbital compounds are best avoided.

Dosage

Dosage is usually one or two pills every 3 hours, as needed. Since the Esgic Plus provides 175 mg of additional acetaminophen, the total amount of acetaminophen needs to be monitored.

Side Effects

Fatigue is a common side effect, as is lightheadedness. Occasionally, nervousness is experienced. Nausea is uncommon. Thus, Esgic is useful for migraine patients for whom nausea is a problem. Since addiction is a major concern, these compounds should not usually be used for daily headaches. In occasional circumstances, however, patients may do very well with one or two Fiorinal or Esgic per day. However, the amounts need to be monitored and limited.

Phrenilin

Phrenilin has the same composition as Esgic but without the caffeine. It contains 50 mg of butalbital and 325 mg of acetaminophen. Although less effective than Fiorinal or Esgic, Phrenilin is helpful for patients who cannot take caffeine or aspirin, and for those who take the medication at night when sleep is desired. Many patients use Fiorinal or Esgic in the morning or afternoon, and Phrenilin at night. Phrenilin Forte is Phrenilin with additional acetaminophen (the same situation as Esgic and Esgic Plus).

Dosage

Dosage is usually one or two pills every 3 hours, as needed.

Side Effects

Fatigue is common since Phrenilin contains no caffeine to offset the butalbital. Otherwise, this medication is usually well tolerated. Lightheadedness may occur, as with all of the butalbital compounds.

Fiorinal with Codeine (Fiorinal #3)

The combination of 30 mg of codeine with Fiorinal is usually more effective than Fiorinal alone, but often produces increased side effects. For patients who tolerate it, Fiorinal with codeine can be a very useful abortive medication. The potential for abuse of this medication is a major concern.

Dosage

Dosage is usually one capsule every 3 hours, or two capsules every 4 hours, as needed.

Side Effects

Fatigue, lightheadedness, and nausea are common, and many patients cannot tolerate codeine. GI upset or abdominal pain are frequent side effects.

Second Line Abortive Therapy

These consist of the following: ergotamine tartrate, DHE injections (or nasal spray), sumatriptan, ketorolac (Toradol) injections, cortisone, and oral narcotics.

We use the second line medications if the first line therapies are not appropriate or effective. In certain patients I will begin treatment with one of the second line abortive medications. If patients are willing to use an injection, DHE or sumatriptan are wise choices. In severe menstrual migraine, cortisone is extremely helpful. A small amount of a narcotic is useful during pregnancy, because we do not have many other choices. In the elderly, narcotics are often utilized in limited doses.

Ergotamine Tartrate

Strong vasoconstrictors, the ergotamines have many limitations, but should be utilized at some point in the treatment of most younger migraine patients. When effective, they stop the migraine, rather than merely cover the pain. The frequent side effects of nausea and nervousness limit use, and the rebound headaches that result from overuse are severe. The very long half-life of ergots contributes to the rebound situation. The most commonly used ergotamine tartrate preparations are Cafergot pills or suppositories and Ergostat sublingual pills. Ergostat pills may be swallowed directly, bypassing the sublingual route. Ergots must be given with caution to patients over 40 years of age because of the increasing risk of myocardial infarction. Peripheral vascular disease or hypertension are contraindications. Ergotamines may exacerbate peptic ulcers. The effective dose of ergotamine varies widely among patients.

Cafergot Pills

Cafergot contains 1 mg of ergotamine tartrate and 100 mg of caffeine. Cafergot pills are the most convenient but least effective of the ergots.

Dosage

Dosage is one or two pills at the onset of headache, repeated every $\frac{1}{2}$ to 1 hour, up to a maximum of five per day and 10 per week. Begin with one pill only in patients who have not used ergots previously. Cafergot must not be used daily, and should be limited to one day in any 4 day period.

Side Effects

Nausea is common, with occasional vomiting as well. If patients are more than mildy nauseated with their migraine, Cafergot is best avoided. Nervousness is a frequent side effect, and, as with any ergot, the anxiety may be severe. The caffeine adds to the nervousness. Insomnia or dizziness may occur. Numbness or tingling in fingers or toes, muscle pain in the extremities, and chest pain may occur but are infrequent. Bradycardia or tachycardia have been reported but are rare. Ergot rebound headaches may result when Cafergot is used 2 or more days consecutively. Cafergot should be used with great caution in patients over 40 years of age because of the potential for coronary artery vasoconstriction. Ergotamines may

---

TABLE 2.2. Quick Reference Guide: Second Line Abortive Migraine Medication.

1. Ergots: Vasoconstrictors with many side effects but usually effective. Nausea and anxiety are common with ergotamine compounds. Cafergot adds caffeine to the ergotamine. Ergostat SL is 2 mg of pure ergotamine. Suppositories are more effective than pills. Rebound headaches are common with overuse of ergots. Use with caution after age 40, particularly with cardiac risk factors.
2. DHE: Effective as an IV or IM injection, and occasionally effective as a nasal spray. DHE is safe and well tolerated. Nausea, leg cramps, and burning at the injection site are common. IV DHE is very effective in the office or emergency room. One mg IM or IV is the usual dose, but this may be titrated up or down.
3. Sumatriptan (Imitrex): Very effective for migraine and cluster headaches. The usual dose is one 100 mg pill (100 mg) orally, or one 6 mg injection (SQ) to start, and this may be repeated in 1 hour. The maximum is two injections or three pills in 24 hours. Forty percent of patients require more than one dose, or another "escape" medication. Nausea or chest pressure are common, as are numbness or taste disturbances. Fatigue and dizziness may also be seen. Side effects are short-lasting. Cost and availablitity are a problem.
4. Ketorolac (Toradol): The injections are much more effective than the pills. Patients may use the injections, 60 mg per 2 cc, at home. The prefilled syringes are easy to use. Usual dose is 60 mg, which may be repeated in 1 hour if necessary. Nausea or GI pain may occur. Ketorolac is nonaddicting and does not usually cause sedation.
5. Corticosteroids: Cortisone is often the most effective therapy for severe, prolonged migraine. Dexamethasone (Decadron) or prednisone are the usual oral forms, and are dosed at 4 mg of Decadron or 20 mg of prednisone every 4 to 6 hours, as needed. Three tablets a month is the usual maximum. These are very helpful for menstrual migraine. The small doses limit side effects, but nausea, anxiety, fatigue, and insomnia are seen.

---

increase arterial blood pressure. Cafergot is usually avoided in patients with hypertension, peripheral vascular disease, or peptic ulcers.

Cafergot Suppositories

Less convenient but much more effective than the pills, Cafergot suppositories contain 2 mg of ergotamine tartrate and 100 mg of caffeine. With patients who are too nauseated to take a pill, Cafergot suppositories are occasionally helpful, but the main side effect to the suppository is nausea itself. The Cafergot PB suppositories (see next section) cause much less nausea and are more effective, but at present Cafergot PB is only available as a generic preparation. Compounding pharmacists can formulate Cafergot PB. (See Table 2.3)

Dosage

Starting with one third or one half of a suppository, the dose is then titrated up or down, depending on the patient's response. The effective dose varies widely among patients. The dose may be repeated after 1 hour, up to a maximum of two suppositories per day and five per week. Use of Cafergot suppositories must be limited to only 1 day in a 4 day

TABLE 2.3. Suppositories, Lozenges, and Nasal Sprays Formulated Through Compounding Pharmacists.

Suppositories: Compounding pharmacists are able to formulate combinations of medications that are not commercially available. For instance, meperidine (Demerol) may be made into a suppository, and Phenergan or Tigan can be added to this. Decadron, which is helpful for severe migraines, may be added to an analgesic and/or an antiemetic, and used as a suppository. The absorption is not very good with Decadron in the rectal mucosa, but some of the medication is absorbed. For patients who are too nauseated for oral medication, the suppository route is one option.

Lozenges: Compounding pharmacists are able to put medication in lozenge form, to be absorbed by the mouth's buccal mucosa. For instance, Phenergan or Tigan may be used for nausea in this fashion. Acetaminophen may be used as a lozenge for children who cannot or will not swallow pills. We do not generally wish to use suppositories in children, and lozenges are one alternative.

Nasal spray: Compounding pharmacists are able to put dihydroergotamine (DHE) in a nasal spray form that is less effective than the IM injections, but much more convenient. The nasal spray of DHE will become commercially available.

period. Some patients find as little as one fifth of a suppository is all that they require.

Side Effects

Side effects of Cafergot suppositories are the same as those of Cafergot pills, except that nausea is slightly less common. Many migraineurs experience diarrhea along with their headaches, and cannot tolerate a suppository.

Cafergot PB Suppositories

More effective than plain Cafergot suppositories, Cafergot PB contains 2 mg of ergotamine tartrate, 100 mg of caffeine, 0.25 mg l-alkaloids of belladonna, and 60 mg of pentobarbital. Dosage is the same as for plain Cafergot suppositories. Side effects are less, with decreased nausea. Sedation may be a problem due to the pentobarbital. The major problem has been availability of the Cafergot PB suppositories; only the generic preparation has been available lately. Compounding pharmacists are extremely valuable in formulating migraine preparations such as Cafergot PB suppositories.

Ergostat Pills

These contain 2 mg of ergotamine tartrate with no caffeine. They may be utilized sublingually, or simply swallowed. The usual dosage is one pill at the onset of the headache that may be repeated after 1 hour. The maximum is two per day and five per week. Side effects are the same as with Cafergot, but less anxiety is seen due to the lack of caffeine.

DHE (Dihydroergotamine)

This compound is different from the other ergots in that it is only a very mild arterial vasoconstrictor; DHE most likely works through serotonergic effects (it is a venoconstrictor). I consider DHE to be safer than the other ergotamines, and I will use DHE in older age ranges if there are no contraindications. Sumatriptan is actually a more selective form of DHE, with somewhat fewer side effects.

DHE is not effective orally, and is usually given as an IM injection. I have been using DHE as a nasal spray, but this is not yet commercially available. Compounding pharmacists formulate the nasal spray from the DHE powder. For patients willing to give themselves an injection, IM DHE is an extremely effective abortive medication. It is also very effective when given intravenously. Rebound headaches are not a problem with DHE, and DHE may be used on 2 consecutive days.

Dosage

One mg (one vial) is the usual dose, but some patients only tolerate $\frac{1}{2}$ mg, and others need $1\frac{1}{2}$ mg. The initial dose of 1 mg may be repeated in 1 hour, if necessary. I use either insulin syringes or 25 gauge 3 cc $\frac{5}{8}$ or 1 inch syringes. Icing the injection site may prevent local pain. Intramuscular DHE is less painful, and slightly more effective, than subcutaneous DHE. DHE is best limited to 2 mg in a day, but it may be used on 2 consecutive days. Unlike the other ergots, DHE does not usually cause rebound headaches when overused or used for several consecutive days. Still, it should be limited to 5 mg in a week. In the emergency room or office, IV administration of DHE is a valuable migraine abortive technique. The nasal spray is formulated by compounding pharmacists, and the usual dose is one spray in each nostril; this may be repeated in 10 minutes. After the second dose, one spray in each nostril may be repeated every 2 hours, as needed, up to a maximum of four sprays in each nostril per day, at most. The nasal spray is also limited to 12 sprays per week at most. The side effects are similar to those of IM DHE, but less severe. However, extreme nasal stuffiness may occur. (See Chapter 3 for a discussion of the IV DHE protocol.)

Side Effects

Nausea is a very common side effect of DHE, and many patients need to be given antinausea medication before the DHE is administered. Reglan, 5 or 10 mg PO, Compazine 5 to 25 mg PO, IM, or as a suppository, Tigan 250 mg PO or as a 200 mg suppository, or Phenergan 25 to 50 mg PO, IM, or as a suppository are typical nausea medications. For home use, it is helpful to have the patient take the nausea medication at least 10 minutes prior to the DHE. When Phenergan is used, it can be used with DHE in

TABLE 2.4. Ergotamines for Migraine.

Name	Composition
Cafergot pills	Ergotamine, 1 mg and caffeine, 100 mg
Cafergot suppositories	Ergotamine, 2 mg, and caffeine, 100 mg
Cafergot PB suppositories (generic may be only form available)	Ergotamine, 2 mg, caffeine, 100 mg, pentobarbital, 60 mg, and 0.25 mg l-alkaloids of belladonna
Ergostat sublingual pills	Ergotamine, 2 mg
Ergotrate (ergonovine)	Ergonovine, 0.2 mg
Bellergal-S tablets	Ergotamine, 0.6 mg, phenobarbital, 40 mg, and belladonna, 0.2 mg
Dihydroergotamine (DHE) injections, nasal spray	DHE, 1 mg per injection, spray is variously formulated
Imitrex (sumatriptan) injections (not a true ergotamine)	Sumatriptan, 6 mg

the same syringe. Many patients experience a flushed feeling of heat in the head. A muscle tension, mild headache may occur briefly. Leg cramps or aching in the legs is common. Numbness or burning may be experienced around the injection site, and this may be prevented by "icing" the injection site prior to administration. Diarrhea is frequently a side effect, particularly with IV administration, and may be treated with Imodium or Lomotil. This is transient, rarely lasting more than 1 day. Tightness in the chest or throat is another common effect, and is either muscular or gastrointestinal in origin. Antacids or Tums are helpful in some patients with heartburn or GI upset due to DHE. All of these side effects tend to be of short duration. Serious side effects are very rare, but angina has been reported several times, and supraventricular tachycardias have been occasionally noted in patients on tricyclic antidepressants given DHE. Vascular compromise in an extremity has been reported in patients given DHE in large amounts. The vascular compromise was reversed by administering calcium blockers. In patients receiving a combination of beta blockers and IV DHE, vascular problems may be somewhat more likely to occur. Generally, DHE has proven to be a safe medication. However, pregnancy, prinzmetal angina, poorly controlled hypertension, and peripheral vascular disease are absolute contraindications.

Sumatriptan (Imitrex) Pills and Injections

Sumatriptan is a serotonin-1 (5-ht-1) receptor agonist, presumably effective because of its ability to decrease neurogenic inflammation in the dura, or due to cranial blood vessel vasoconstriction. Sumatriptan is possibly the most effective antimigraine abortive agent. The pills and injections are both effective, and side effects tend to be minimal. The cost of sumatriptan is very high, and availability of the oral form in the United States has been difficult; at the time of this publication, the oral form of sumatriptan has not been released for use in the United States. Sumatriptan has a short half-life of about 2 hours, and thus recurrence of the migraine happens in approximately 40% of patients. This occurs within 12 to 24 hours of the resolution of the initial migraine symptoms. The self-injector unit used with sumatriptan is very convenient.

Relief with sumatriptan is rapid, particularly with the subcutaneous injections. Clinical response is usually seen within 10 to 15 minutes following subcutaneous administration, and within 30 minutes for the oral form. Escape pain medications are often needed after the sumatriptan has ceased working. Vasoconstrictors (Ergotamines, Midrin) should not be utilized until at least 6 hours after sumatriptan administration. Sumatriptan cannot be used with MAOI's. Sumatriptan should not be used until at least 24 hours after ergotamine use, and at least 6 hours after Midrin. Sumatriptan is very expensive; approximate cost to the patient in the United States is 35 dollars per injection, and 18 dollars per pill. Rebound headache may occur, but this has been less of a problem than with older ergots.

Dosage

The injectable dosage is one 6 mg injection at the onset, and then one more may be repeated, at least 1 hour after the first. The injection is subcutaneous, not intramuscular. Two injections is the maximum dose per 24 hours.

The usual dose of the tablets is one of the 100 mg pills at the onset. Within 2 hours, 50% to 75% of patients have obtained relief, and by 4 hours another 15% to 25% have had relief of the headache. If there is no response within 4 hours, the sumatriptan is usually not further utilized, and escape pain medication is used. If the sumatriptan is not effective for one attack, it may still be utilized for future migraines. If the sumatriptan does help, but the pain recurs, an additional oral 100 mg dose may be given, up to a maximum of 300 mg (3 tablets) per 24 hours. Because this is a new drug, we do not as yet know the effects of overuse of sumatriptan. Until further studies, and time, reveal otherwise, limits of four pills or injections per week should be imposed. Analgesics and anti-emetics may be utilized concurrently with sumatriptan.

Side Effects

The side effects of sumatriptan are generally less than with DHE. Most side effects resolve within 10 to 30 minutes. Transient pain at the injection site is common, as is seen with DHE; "icing" the injection site prior to administration may prevent this. Nausea is relatively common, but sumatriptan (and DHE) often actually decrease the nausea of a migraine. Taste disturbances, fatigue, and dizziness are also seen relatively frequently. Tingling sensations in the extremities are common and transient.

Heat flashes, and feelings of pressure or heaviness may be experienced in any part of the body. Chest pain and heaviness are commonly experienced. Flushing and feelings of weakness may occur. Minor transient increases in the blood pressure have been seen. Sumatriptan should not be used in pregnant women, children or adolescents, women who are nursing, patients with hepatic or renal impairment, or with cardiovascular disease. Patients over the age of 45 should be screened for cardiac risk factors, and sumatriptan has not been approved for use after age 65. The etiology of the chest pressure or discomfort seen with sumatriptan is unknown, but may be related to stretch receptors in pulmonary vasculature.

Ketorolac (Toradol) Injections (IM)

Ketorolac is useful as a migraine abortive, particularly when oral medication cannot be utilized. It is well tolerated, and patients can learn to self-administer the injections at home. Ketorolac is only mild to moderately effective, but the lack of sedation or addiction potential renders it very important in office or emergency room management of acute migraines.

Dosage

Ketorolac is available as a 30 mg per cc injection, or as 60 mg per 2 cc in prefilled syringes. The usual dose is 60 mg, that may then be repeated as another 30 or 60 mg in 1 hour. The maximum is 120 mg per day, and I recommend only using ketorolac once or twice per week as an injection. The total dose per week and per month needs to be monitored because of the possible renal, GI, or hepatic toxicity.

Side Effects

GI upset or GI pain occur frequently, as ketorolac is a nonsteroidal anti-inflammatory. Sedation is infrequent but does occur. Hepatic and renal functions need to be monitored, and ketorolac should not be given in the face of hepatic or renal impairment.

Corticosteroids

Cortisone, used judiciously in limited amounts, is often the only effective therapy for severe, prolonged migraine. It is usually given PO or IM. Menstrual migraines that are refractive to standard migraine therapy may respond particularly well to cortisone (see Chapter 4 on menstrual migraine). Cortisone is an effective preventive therapy for altitude and flying headaches. Dexamethasone (Decadron) or prednisone may be used for oral administration, and Depo-Medrol or ACTH for IM use. Dexamethasone is probably the most effective oral preparation.

Dosage

Dosage is usually one 20 mg prednisone or one 4 mg Decadron tablet taken with food and repeated as needed every 4 to 6 hours. If side effects occur, the dose may be dropped to one-half pill with each dose, I limit the cortisone to a maximum of three tablets per month; of course, in any one month, more than three tablets would not usually present a problem, but it is important to set guidelines for patients and emphasize the limits of this medication. Because cortisone is extremely effective for certain patients, if given access to large numbers of pills, they may overuse the Decadron or prednisone.

For flying headaches one half or one pill of Decadron or prednisone is taken approximately $\frac{1}{2}$ hour prior to the flight, and $\frac{1}{2}$ or one pill may be repeated.

For altitude migraines, one pill is taken prior to arrival, and then one half or one pill is repeated after arrival. This may need to be repeated in the first 2 days.

For severe, prolonged migraine, 40 to 80 mg of Depo-Medrol IM, or 40 to 80 units of ACTH gel IM may be given, but must be limited to once per 2 months at most. Anecdotal evidence indicates that the ACTH gel is somewhat more effective than the Depo-Medrol. If nausea precludes the use of cortisone pills, compounding pharmacists can formulate oral lozenges or rectal suppositories of dexamethasone, and this may be combined with antiemetic and analgesic medication.

Side Effects

In the limited amounts used for migraine, steroids very rarely produce severe side effects. Even though they are being used in small doses for short bursts of time, patients need to be aware of the potential side effects. Short term side effects include nausea, insomnia, GI upset, nervousness, and facial flushing. Weight gain or water retention may occur. Fatigue can be a problem, as can agitation. Very rarely, femoral head necrosis has been reported, even with small amounts of steroids. In general, however, steroids are well tolerated over the short term.

Narcotics and Sedatives

When the usual first line medications do not help, stronger narcotics may be given PO or IM, usually with antinausea medication at the same time. The nausea, and their potential for causing addiction, limit their usefulness. These medications often help calm the patient and induce sleep. The narcotics are useful for the short term (1 to 3 days). They should not be utilized on a daily basis except where every other method for controlling daily headaches has failed. In these unusual circumstances, patients need to limit use to small amounts of a daily narcotic. Besides the addiction potential, all of the narcotics can cause fatigue, stomach upset or pain, and nausea. Many patients become euphoric, or experience a relief of anxiety or depression. These effects are very short lived. Constipation may be a problem for some patients. There are a number of headache patients where only sedatives or narcotics are effective.

The milder narcotics are oral preparations. Fiorinal #3 (mentioned earlier in this chapter) is very helpful because it contains aspirin, caffeine, butalbital, and 30 mg of codeine. All of these ingredients are helpful for migraine. Acetaminophen with codeine preparations (Tylenol #3, Tylenol #4) do not contain aspirin, and therefore induce less nausea. Aspirin and codeine (Empirin with codeine) is somewhat more effective than codeine and acetaminophen, because aspirin is more effective for migraine than acetaminophen. However, the aspirin may induce more nausea. Hydrocodone with acetaminophen (Vicodin and Lorcet) is a well tolerated narcotic preparation. Propoxyphene (Darvon or Darvocet) has been helpful for some patients. The usual dose of the narcotics is one or two pills every 3 or 4 hours, as needed.

The stronger narcotics include meperidine (Demerol), methadone (Dolophine), oxycodone (Percocet, Percodan, Tylox), and morphine. For some patients, these medications provide the only relief that they may have from their severe migraines. Methadone has certain advantages over meperidine, as it is longer lasting, slightly less apt to cause addiction, and less likely to induce nausea. The usual dose of oral meperidine is 50 to 100 mg every 3 to 4 hours, as needed. Methadone is dosed at 5 or 10 mg every 3 to 4 hours, oxycodone is one tablet every 3 to 4 hours, and morphine is one 15 mg tablet every 3 to 4 hours. Limits of three or four tablets per day, at most, must be established. Monthly limits of the stronger narcotics, usually at 10 pills per month at most, need to be established with the patients. A prescription for 30 pills every 3 months is reasonable; more than this should be avoided, except in very unusual circumstances.

The injections of the above narcotics are, of course, much more effective. Demerol is dosed at 50 to 125 mg per injection; methadone at 5 to 10 mg; and morphine at 10 to 15 mg. The addition of a nausea medication with the injection is very helpful, for it potentiates the narcotic and is sedating for the patient. The antiemetic medication also aids the nausea of the migraine, and also offsets the nausea induced by the narcotic. Demerol or morphine may be formulated by a compounding pharmacist as an oral lozenge or a rectal suppository, and this may be combined with antiemetic medication in the same preparation.

Sedatives helpful in the acute treatment of migraine include the butalbital medications (see section on butalbital medications), the antiemetics (see next section on antinausea medication), and the benzodiazepines. Sedation is always useful for severe migraine, as sleep is a powerful weapon against the headache. Benzodiazepines include diazepam (Valium) and clonazepam (Klonopin).

Valium is preferable over its generic, diazepam. Valium's sedative and muscle relaxant properties aid in treating the migraine pain and associated muscle contraction. The dose is 5 or 10 mg, repeated every 3 to 4 hours if necessary. Valium should be limited to 20 mg per day at most. Sedation is common, as is euphoria. Valium should not be used on a daily basis, except in unusual circumstances.

Klonopin is useful in some patients, probably because of its strong sedative effects. Klonopin is occasionally useful in treating patients with daily headaches, particularly when insomnia is present. It is best, however, to try and avoid daily use of the benzodiazepines. Klonopin is dosed at 0.5 to 2 mg every 3 to 4 hours, as needed, with a maximum of 4 mg per day at most.

Intravenous Prochlorperazine (Compazine)

Intravenous Compazine is very effective for severe nausea, and it will often stop the pain of the migraine as well. Compazine may be given for both the pain and nausea of the migraine attack. In the emergency room or hospital, this drug may be given prior to DHE. If the pain of the migraine is much improved after the intravenous compazine, I will usually forego giving the DHE, and simply wait to see if the migraine pain returns. Intravenous Compazine is very sedating, and this is usually helpful for the migraineur. Severe anxiety or restlessness may occur with IV Compazine, and is a very distressing reaction.

Dosage

The Compazine is given intravenously as a 5 or 10 mg dose. The first time the patient has been given IV Compazine, I will only give 5 mg, and observe the response. If a patient is known to tolerate it well, 10 mg may be given in one dose. If 10 mg is not sufficient, I will abandon the Compazine, and utilize DHE, sumatriptan, Toradol, or narcotics.

Side Effects

Inner restlessness and anxiety are seen occasionally with IV Compazine, and this side effect is often extremely upsetting to the patient. Benzodiazepines are helpful in countering this effect. Sedation is common with the intravenous Compazine, and this often will allow the migraineur to sleep, which decreases the pain of the attack. Hypotension may occur, and fluids may then be given intravenously. An intravenous line should be utilized for the IV Compazine treatment. Extrapyramidal side effects may occur, and diphenhydramine (Benadryl) is helpful for this situation. The diphenhydramine is given in the dosage of 25 to 50 mg IV or deeply IM; rarely, doses of 100 mg may be required. This may be repeated, up to a maximum of 400 mg per day.

Antiemetic Medication

If patients have pills or suppositories of antinausea medication on hand, they are often able to avoid an emergency room trip. Most of the antinausea medications are sedating, which is usually felt by migraineurs to be helpful. Rectal suppositories are less convenient than pills but are more effective. The antiemetics may cause hypotension. If suppositories have failed to give relief, patients with severe nausea and vomiting may self-administer IM injections of antinausea medication. Most patients with severe nausea find it convenient to keep both the pills and suppositories available.

Promethazine (Phenergan)

Promethazine, a mild antinausea medication, has certain advantages: it has an extremely low incidence of extrapyramidal side effects, is safe in children, and is sedating.

Dosage

Dosage is usually 25 to 50 mg PO every 3 to 4 hours as needed. The 25 or 50 mg suppositories also are very effective. In patients who have become overly fatigued by the 25 mg dose, half of a 25 mg tablet, or one 12.5 mg tablet, may be prescribed. As an IM injection, promethazine may be mixed in the same syringe with a narcotic or with DHE-45.

TABLE 2.5. Quick Reference Guide: Antiemetic Medication.

1. Promethazine (Phenergan): Mild but effective for most patients. Very sedating. Low incidence of extrapyramidal side effects. Available as pills, suppositories, and oral lozenges (formulated by compounding pharmacists). Used for children and adults.
2. Prochlorperazine (Compazine): Very effective but high incidence of extrapyramidal side effects. Anxiety and agitation are common. Given intravenously, it may stop the migraine pain as well as the nausea. Pills, long acting spansules, and suppositories are available.
3. Metoclopramide (Reglan): Mild but well tolerated, commonly used prior to IV DHE. Fatigue or anxiety occur but are not usually severe. Five to 10 mg are given PO, IM, or IV.
4. Trimethobenzamide (Tigan): Well tolerated, useful in children and adults. Pills, suppositories, or oral lozenges may be used (lozenges formulated by compounding pharmacists).
5. Chlorpromazine (Thorazine): Extremely effective but with increased side effects, particularly sedation. The suppositories often prevent an ER trip by sedating the patient and stopping the nausea. Used with patients where other antiemetics have failed.

Side Effects

Fatigue is the most common side effect, but this is often beneficial for patients with severe migraine. The extrapyramidal side effects and nervousness caused by other antiemetics are rarely seen with promethazine. Dizziness may occur. Occasionally, hypotension is encountered as a side effect.

Prochlorperazine (Compazine)

Although prochlorperazine is more effective than promethazine, it carries a relatively high incidence of extrapyramidal side effects and anxiety. An inner restlessness may be severe, particularly with IV administration. Most patients do not become heavily sedated by prochlorperazine. In the emergency room, IM or IV prochlorperazine not only relieves the patient's nausea, but the pain may be improved. (See the previous section on IV prochlorperazine.)

Dosage

Dosage is usually 10 to 25 mg PO every 3 to 4 hours, with a maximum of 60 mg per day. Suppositories (5 or 25 mg) are very useful. The usual IM or IV dose is 5 or 10 mg. Long-acting oral spansules (10, 15, and 30 mg) are available and may be dosed at 6 hour intervals.

Side Effects

Side effects of anxiety, agitation, and extrapyramidal effects occur more commonly with prochlorperazine than with promethazine. Hypotension may occur, particularly with IV administration. Fatigue may occur but is not usually a problem. Although these side effects are relatively common, for the patients who tolerate the drug, it is usually very effective.

Metoclopramide (Reglan)

A mild antinausea medication, metoclopramide carries a low incidence of side effects. Fatigue is common but tends to be mild. Usually given as 10 mg tablets, metoclopramide is also useful intramuscularly or intravenously.

Dosage

Dosage is 5 or 10 mg every 4 hours, as needed, up to a maximum of 30 mg per day. Used as a premedication prior to IV administration of DHE, metoclopramide may be given as 5 or 10 mg PO or IV. (See Chapter 3 for the IV DHE protocol.)

Side Effects

Restlessness and fatigue may occur, but are usually mild. Extrapyramidal side effects are occasionally encountered. Generally, metoclopramide is very well tolerated.

Trimethobenzamide (Tigan)

Although Tigan may be somewhat less effective than the strongest antiemetics, it is usually extremely well tolerated. Tigan is a useful medication for children.

Dosage

250 mg PO or 200 mg as a suppository is the usual dose, taken every 3 hours as needed. Tigan is also available for IM use.

Side Effects

Side effects are minimal with Tigan. Fatigue may occur but is not common. Extrapyramidal side effects are occasionally seen, as is hypotension. Anxiety or restlessness occur much less frequently than with prochlorperazine.

Chlorpromazine (Thorazine)

Chlorpromazine is the most effective antinausea agent. The 100 mg suppositories are very effective and sedating. Chlorpromazine appears to relieve the pain of migraine as well as the nausea. For patients who are subject to the most severe migraines, having available a combination of a strong narcotic and chlorpromazine often allows them to manage their headaches at home. Side effects are more frequent with chlorpromazine than with the milder antinausea medications.

Dosage

Dosage is usually 25 to 50 mg PO or as a suppository, every 3 hours, as needed. Tablets are available in 10, 25, 50, 100, and 200 mg sizes. Suppositories are available in 25 and 100 mg sizes. The 100 mg suppositories may be cut in half. The 100 mg suppositories, although very sedating, are useful for those patients who experience severe, prolonged vomiting.

Side Effects

Sedation is common, long-lasting, and often severe. Extrapyramidal side effects occur occasionally. Extreme dizziness may be seen. Some patients, particularly those on higher doses, become almost incoherent because of slurred speech and severe sedation. In lower doses, however, most patients tolerate Thorazine fairly well.

CHAPTER 3

Migraine Preventive Medication

First Line Preventive Medication

Preventive therapy is useful when patients experience more than three moderate to severe headaches per month, or if the abortive medications have not provided sufficient relief. It is an individual decision based upon the person's willingness to take daily medications, the severity of the headaches, and how much the patient is bothered by the migraine situation. By utilizing daily preventive medicine, patients actually ingest less overall medication because they are not constantly chasing after the headaches with analgesics. The goal of preventive therapy is to decrease the number of migraines by at least 50% to 90% and to lessen the severity of the pain. Patients must realize that we are simply attempting to decrease the overall impact of their migraine headaches, not completely eliminate them. It would be outstanding if the preventive medication completely stopped the headaches from occurring, but this is not realistic with most patients. A compromise must be struck between overmedicating the patient and the number of migraines they suffer; to add more preventive medication in order to eliminate one more migraine every 2 months is usually not worthwhile.

Many of the medications used for migraine have not received specific FDA indications for this use. The following is only a guide to what I consider reasonable and rational therapy for headache; prior to prescribing medications for patients, they need to be informed of, and accept, the complete set of contraindications and side effects as listed in the PDR and package insert.

The choice of first line preventive medication must be tailored to individual patients and depends upon whether they suffer also from chronic tension headaches. Important considerations include age, sleeping pattern, gastrointestinal or other medical problems, blood pressure, and pulse.

First line choices for preventing migraine involve four classes of medication: (1) antidepressants, (2) beta blockers, (3) anti-inflammatories, and (4) calcium blockers.

TABLE 3.1. Criteria for the Use of Preventive Medication.

1. More than 3 moderate or severe headaches per month.
2. Abortive medications have failed to provide sufficient relief.
3. Quality of life is significantly decreased due to the migraine severity or frequency.
4. The patient is willing to take daily medication, endure possible side effects, and change medications, if necessary.

TABLE 3.2. Quick Reference Guide: First Line Preventive Medication for Migraine.

1. Amitriptyline (Elavil): Effective, inexpensive, and also useful for daily headaches and insomnia. Use in low doses, at night, Sedation, weight gain, dry mouth, and constipation are common. Starting dose is 10 mg, working up to 25 or 50 mg; can be pushed to 200 mg, or decreased to 5 mg.
2. Propranolol (Inderal): Effective. Long acting (LA) capsules may be dosed once per day. Occasionally effective for daily headaches. Sedation, diarrhea, lower GI upset, and weight gain are common. Very useful in combination with amitriptyline. Dosage begins with the LA 60 mg, and is usually kept between 60 and 160 mg per day.
3. Naproxen (Naprosyn, Anaprox): Useful in younger patients, once a day dosing. Sometimes helpful for daily headaches. Particularly useful for menstrual migraine. Nonsedating, but frequent GI upset. Effective as an abortive, and may be combined with other first line preventive medications. The usual dose is 500 or 550 mg once a day, but this may be pushed to twice a day.
4. Verapamil: Reasonably effective for migraine, once a day dosing with the slow release (SR) tablets. Usually nonsedating, and weight gain is uncommon. Occasionally helpful for daily headaches. May be combined with other first line medications, particularly amitriptyline or naproxen. Constipation is common. Starting dose is one half of a 240 mg SR pill, increasing quickly to one 240 mg pill per day. May be pushed to 240 mg twice a day, or decreased to 120 mg or 180 mg per day.

Antidepressants

This class of medication is very useful as a first line migraine preventive. Antidepressants are particularly helpful when daily tension headaches are present. The antimigraine effect is separate from the antidepressant effect, and the doses used for migraine patients are usually subtherapeutic for depression. The most effective tricyclic antidepressant is amitriptyline. The monoamine oxidase inhibitors (MAOI) are extremely effective for migraine and are discussed in the section on third line preventives.

Amitriptyline (Elavil)

Amitriptyline is the most commonly used, least expensive, and most effective of the tricyclic antidepressants. Both migraine and daily headaches respond well, and amitriptyline also improves sleep. Inexpensive for daily use, this medication is particularly helpful for patients who have both migraine and chronic tension headaches.

Dosage

Amitriptyline is usually started at 10 mg taken each night, and this is slowly increased over several weeks to 50 mg. Because of its sedative effect, amitriptyline is ordinarily used only at night, but occasionally patients do better with split doses throughout the day. If excessive early morning sedation occurs, taking the medication earlier in the evening, at 7 or 8 p.m., may help. Beginning with too high a dose severely decreases the likelihood that patients will comply, but if patients can stay on amitriptyline for any length of time, the sedative effects usually decrease to a tolerable level. Most patients do well with low amounts, some with as little as 5 mg (one half of a 10 mg pill). If needed, the dose may be pushed to 150 or 200 mg, but if these doses are ineffective, higher doses usually will not help. As with any preventive medication, 4 weeks should be allowed for a trial period before abandoning that drug.

Side Effects

Sedation, weight gain, and constipation are the major limiting side effects. (See Table 3.3) These can usually be minimized by lowering the dose. Dry mouth and dizziness are common. Oral balance gel and Biotene toothpaste are OTC preparations useful for dry mouth. Anxiety or nervousness may initially occur, but these feelings are usually transient. Depression, blurred vision, memory difficulties, and insomnia also may occur.

Tachycardia may be a problem, and is often the limiting factor on increasing the dose. A beta blocker may be prescribed additionally for both migraine prevention and for the tachycardia.

Fluoxetine (Prozac)

Fluoxetine is an antidepressant that has been effective in certain migraine patients, and has a favorable side effect profile. Fluoxetine is a selective

TABLE 3.3. Antidepressants: Sedation and Weight Gain.

Drug	Sedation	Weight Gain
Doxepin (Sinequan)	Severe	Severe
Amitriptyline (Elavil)	Severe	Severe
Protriptyline (Vivactil)	None	None
Fluoxetine (Prozac)	Mild	Mild
Sertraline (Zoloft)	Mild	Mild
Nortriptyline (Pamelor)	Moderate	Moderate
Desipramine (Norpramin)	Mild	Mild
Trimipramine (Surmontil)	Severe	Severe
Phenelzine (Nardil)	Mild	Very severe

serotonin reuptake inhibitor that is the first of what will be many similar medications. Sertraline (Zoloft) is a new serotonin reuptake inhibitor that is very much like fluoxetine, but with somewhat less side effects. Sertraline will possibly be increasingly used for headache, and is discussed in this chapter under miscellaneous antidepressants, and also in Chapter 7. The absence of weight gain and the lack of sedation are major advantages for many patients. Like amitriptyline, fluoxetine is useful for patients who have both chronic tension headaches and migraine headaches. Fluoxetine is also extremely effective for depression, particularly chronic low level depressions. Anxiety and panic attacks are also treated with fluoxetine.

The previous controversy over fluoxetine has abated, and it has proven to be a relatively safe medication. In clinical trials fluoxetine has not increased suicide or violent behavior. Fluoxetine is an expensive medication for daily use.

Dosage

Fluoxetine is available as a 10 or 20 mg capsule, and the beginning dosage is 10 mg each morning. This is raised, after 4 days, to 20 mg each morning. Liquid Prozac is also available, 20 mg per 5 cc. Occasionally, 5 or 10 mg a day is effective. To use one-half capsule per day, have the patient dissolve one capsule in juice, then drink half of the juice each of two days. The dose may be increased to four capsules a day.

Fluoxetine may be combined with amitriptyline (fluoxetine in the morning, amitriptyline at night). However, administration of fluoxetine with tricyclics has resulted in increased blood tricyclic concentrations. Fluoxetine has a very long half-life, 1 to 3 days for the parent compound and 7 to 9 days for the metabolite. This is an expensive medication to use on a daily basis.

Side Effects

Nausea, anxiety or agitation, insomnia, and tremulousness are common. Fatigue and weight gain are much less common than with most antidepressants, but occasionally occur. Weight loss and decreased appetite usually do not occur until higher doses (3 or 4 pills per day) are used. Liver functions must be monitored, since they occasionally elevate with the use of fluoxetine, as with any antidepressant. Decreased WBCs and RBCs are rarely due to the antidepressants but a CBC must be done routinely. Cardiac side effects are rare, but bradycardia or tachycardia may occur.

Doxepin (Sinequan)

Very similar to amitriptyline, doxepin is extremely helpful with migraines, tension headaches, and anxiety. Sedation and weight gain are common, however.

Dosage

Starting dose is 10 mg per day and is slowly increased to 50 or 75 mg. The dose may be increased to 150 mg or more, but generally, if 150 mg is not effective, the medication should be changed. Because of sedation, doxepin is usually only given at night.

Side Effects

Side effects are similar to amitriptyline, with sedation, weight gain, dry mouth, dizziness, and constipation being the primary problems. (See section on side effects of amitriptyline.)

Miscellaneous Antidepressants

Except for the MAO inhibitors (see section on third line prevention medication) most antidepressants, other than those listed above, have been only mildly effective for migraine. They are more useful in chronic daily headache. Trazodone (Desyrel) has been used extensively with little success. Nortriptyline is occasionally helpful in migraine, as is protriptyline (Vivactil). A new serotonin reuptake inhibitor, sertraline (Zoloft), is helpful for some patients with migraine or tension headaches. Sertraline is well tolerated, with much fewer side effects than the older antidepressants.

Nortriptyline (Pamelor, Aventyl)

Nortriptyline, a metabolite of amitriptyline, is usually better tolerated than amitriptyline, causing less sedation. Nortriptyline is used for migraines in patients where amitriptyline has been effective but side effects too severe. Because of the low incidence of cardiac side effects, nortriptyline is the safest tricyclic antidepressant to use for elderly patients. Nortriptyline is more expensive and less effective than amitriptyline. However, it is now available as a generic. As with the other antidepressants, nortriptyline is helpful with chronic tension headaches, and with anxiety.

Dosage

Doses begin at 10 mg, and are slowly increased to 50 to 100 mg, ordinarily taken at night.

Side Effects

Side effects are similar to those of amitriptyline, but less severe. The sedation, dry mouth, weight gain, dizziness, and constipation occur with some patients, but these problems are usually less than with amitriptyline. Tachycardia is not as pronounced as with amitriptyline, but may limit the dose.

Protriptyline (Vivactil)

Proptriptyline is not sedating, does not cause weight gain, and is occasionally helpful in migraine. It is more useful in tension headache. There are patients who respond well to protriptyline for both their migraine and tension headaches. Although anticholinergic side effects may be severe, the absence of weight gain or fatigue are major advantages. For a discussion of protriptyline, please see the section on protriptyline in Chapter 7.

Sertraline (Zoloft)

Sertraline is a relatively new serotonin reuptake inhibitor, much like fluoxetine. It has only recently been used for migraine or tension headache, but early results are promising for both types of headache. Like fluoxetine, sertraline may be used in conjunction with tricyclics, but increased tricyclic levels may result. Sertraline has a shorter half-life than fluoxetine. The parent compound of sertraline and its metabolite have a half-life of 1 day and 3 to 4 days, respectively; fluoxetine's is 1 to 3 days for the parent compound, and 7 to 9 for the metabolite. The lack of weight gain and sedation are a distinct advantage for sertraline over the older tricyclics, and the anticholinergic side effects are less. Sertraline is an effective antidepressant.

Dosage

Sertraline is available in 50 and 100 mg scored tablets. The scored tablets render dosage adjustments easy, which is difficult with fluoxetine. Sertraline is started with one half of a 50 mg tablet, increasing to one tablet in 4 days. The dose may then be pushed to 100, 150, or even 200 mg. For depression, the dose varies widely, between 25 and 200 mg per day. Sertraline should be administered once daily, either in the morning or evening. Sertraline is expensive, and using the 100 mg tablets is less expensive than working with the 50 mg; one half of a 100 mg tablet is cheaper than one 50 mg tablet.

Side Effects

The side effects of sertraline are similar to those of fluoxetine, with nausea, diarrhea, headache, dry mouth, fatigue, dizziness, tremor, insomnia, sexual dysfunction, constipation, or increased sweating occurring in between 8% and 21% of patients. Anxiety or nervousness may also be a problem. Sertraline is, in general, very well tolerated.

Beta-Adrenergic Blocking Agents

Medications in this group are as effective as amitriptyline, and along with amitriptyline they form the backbone of migraine prevention. Because

TABLE **3.4.** Information for Patients Prior to Starting Prevention Medication.

1. The realistic goals of the medication are to decrease the migraine intensity and/or severity by 70%, not to completely eliminate the headaches. It is excellent when the headaches are 90% to 100% improved, but the idea is to minimize medication. Most patients need to be willing to settle for moderate improvement.
2. Patients must be willing to change medication, if necessary. They need to know that what works for somebody else may not work for them, and the first preventive medication chosen may not be effective.
3. Side effects are possible with any medication, and the patient needs to be willing to endure mild side effects in order to achieve results. We cannot simply stop medication and switch to another because of very mild side effects. Most patients are very willing to tolerate mild, annoying side effects.
4. The prevention medication may take weeks to become effective, the doses may need to be adjusted, and they will need patience with the medications. The physician should be available for phone consultations pertaining to the headaches and medicine.
5. Most migraine preventive medications are utilized for other conditions in medicine. Patients need to know what condition the medication is used for other than headache; for example, it helps very much if patients are aware that Prozac is an antidepressant, and that we are using Prozac not because they are depressed, but because of its effects on serotonin.

TABLE **3.5.** Beta-Adrenergic Blocking Agents in Migraine.

Name	Cardioselectivity	Penetration into CNS
Nadolol	No	Low
Timolol	No	Low to medium
Propranolol	No	High
Atenolol	Yes	Low
Metoprolol	Yes	Medium

they lower the pulse, beta blockers are very useful in combination with antidepressants, which often cause a tachycardia. The antianxiety effect of beta blockers is helpful for selected patients. The various medications in this class differ in their mechanism of action and in their efficacy in migraine, and if the first choice has failed, it is often worthwhile to try another. The mainstay of this group remains the original beta blocker used in migraine, propranolol (Inderal). (See Table 3.5)

Propranolol (Inderal)

Propranolol has been extensively used and studied in migraine prophylaxis. The antianxiety effects are useful for some patients, and propranolol is occasionally effective in tension headache as well as for migraine.

Dosage

Propranolol is usually started at 60 mg per day using Inderal LA capsules, and titrating up to 80 or 160 mg daily. The vast majority of patients receive maximum benefit by taking between 60 and 160 mg per day, but lower or higher dosages are sometimes useful. The LA capsules are available in 60, 80, 120, and 160 mg dosages. The disadvantage of this LA preparation is that, being a capsule, it is not easily divided, thus making small titrations in dosage difficult. Occasional patients do better taking smaller doses of the regular tablets two to three times a day. Propranolol must be tapered when discontinuing therapy, unless a young person has used it only for a short period of time. It is possible that the regular tablets are more effective than the long acting preparation.

Side Effects

Fatigue and GI upset, particularly diarrhea and flatulence, are common. Insomnia, depression, lightheadedness, and difficulty concentrating also occur fairly often. Decreased exercise tolerance may occur. Weight gain may be a problem. Bradycardia and hypotension may occur but the bradycardia can be an advantage when propranolol is used in combination with amitriptyline. Wheezing may occur even in patients with no history of asthma. Asthma and congestive heart failure are absolute contraindications. In the presence of Raynaud's phenomenon, propranolol must be used with caution. Since CNS penetration is good, the CNS side effects are greater with this drug than with such hydrophilic drugs as atenolol (Tenormin) or nadolol (Corgard). Patients often complain of being "slowed down" with beta blockers. Beta blockers do not usually increase preexisting depression; when they cause depression, it is usually in patients who are not depressed to begin with.

Metoprolol (Lopressor)

Metoprolol is a cardioselective beta blocker. Although not extensively studied for this purpose, it has been useful for migraine and occasionally is effective where propranolol has failed. As with most beta blockers, metoprolol may be beneficial for chronic daily headache.

Dosage

Metoprolol is usually used twice a day, beginning with 25 mg (one half of a 50 mg tablet), and increasing over 10 days to 50 mg (1 tablet) once or twice a day. Increasing the dosage very gradually minimizes side effects and increases patients' compliance. The scored tablet renders it easy to titrate doses, which is an advantage over the propranolol LA capsules. Metoprolol is available in 50 and 100 mg tablets.

Side Effects

Side effects are essentially the same as for propranolol, with fewer respiratory problems.

Nadolol (Corgard)

Nadolol is as effective as propranolol, and has certain advantages. The decreased lipid solubility of nadolol leads to fewer CNS side effects, particularly fatigue. Some patients respond to nadolol who do not respond to propranolol. If one does not help, it is always worthwhile to consider substituting another beta blocker.

Dosage

The scored tablets and once-a-day dosages allow for easy adjustments in the dose. Starting with 40 mg tablets, one-half tablet is used initially. The dosage can be increased to 40 to 120 mg per day. The average effective dose is 80 mg, but many patients do well on as little as 20 mg per day. The scored tablets are available in 20, 40, and 80 mg.

Side Effects

Nadolol has fewer CNS side effects than propranolol, but otherwise, contraindications and side effects are essentially the same as with propranolol.

Atenolol (Tenormin)

Cardioselectivity and decreased CNS penetration are advantages of atenolol. Occasionally, patients who do not respond to the other beta blockers do well with atenolol.

Dosage

Starting with the 50 mg tablet once a day, the dosage may be increased over 7 days to 100 mg per day. The tablets allow easy adjustments in dosage. The average dose is 100 mg.

Side Effects

Because of its cardioselectivity, atenolol has fewer pulmonary side effects than propranolol. However, it needs to be used with extreme caution in patients with even the slightest tendency towards asthma. The decreased CNS penetration leads to less sedation and fewer CNS side effects.

Timolol (Blocadren)

Timolol possesses essentially the same side effects as propranolol. It is sometimes effective for patients where other beta blockers have failed.

Dosage

Twice daily doses are necessary. To minimize side effects, timolol is initiated with a small dose, such as one half of a 10 mg tablet twice a day.

This is increased over 1 week to 10 mg twice a day, and then up to 30 mg twice a day, if necessary. The average daily dose is 20 to 30 mg.

Side Effects

The side effect profile of timolol is very similar to that of propranolol, with essentially the same incidence of CNS side effects.

Nonsteroidal Anti-inflammatories (NSAIDs)

The NSAIDs can be very effective for migraine prophylaxis, but their use is limited by GI, liver, and renal side effects. Because of these side effects, amitriptyline and the beta blockers are usually chosen first. However, the NSAIDs play a major role for migraine in younger patients. The absence of CNS side effects is helpful for those patients who are very sensitive to the sedative properties of the antidepressants and beta blockers. For patients with arthritic or musculoskeletal problems, NSAIDs may serve a dual purpose. They are also particularly useful for menstrual migraine and menstrual cramps. If initially given for abortive therapy, the NSAIDs may be switched to daily use as preventive medication. NSAIDs are expensive. Of the various medications in this class, naproxen has been the most frequently studied for migraine, and the most widely prescribed.

Naproxen (Naprosyn, Anaprox)

Both naproxen (Naprosyn) and its sodium salt (Anaprox) are used for migraine prevention. Anaprox is more rapidly absorbed and is therefore preferred for abortive treatment. Anaprox is often given initially as an abortive along with a preventive such as amitriptyline, and then, at some point in therapy, the Anaprox is utilized daily as a preventive. This is expensive medication when used daily.

Dosage

Naproxen is usually started as a once-a-day dose of 500 mg Naprosyn or 550 mg Anaprox DS taken with the largest meal. The dose may be increased to one pill twice a day (1,000 mg of Naprosyn or 1,100 mg of Anaprox DS). These drugs are always taken with food. Higher doses may be more effective but are not recommended.

Side Effects

Irritation of the GI tract is common with naproxen. If this side effect occurs in cases where naproxen is very effective, one sucralfate (Carafate) pill taken with liquid $\frac{1}{2}$ to 1 hour prior to the naproxen may eliminate the problem. Alternatively, cimetidine (Tagamet) may be helpful. Cytotec is very effective for protecting the GI tract from the NSAIDs, but adds side effects of its own. Treating the side effects of one medication with another is not generally advocated, but, with selected patients, when other approaches have failed, there is a place for this tactic.

Hepatic irritation may occur, and liver functions must be monitored regularly. Blood tests for renal functions need to be drawn, as nephrotoxicity may be a problem. Skin rashes, fatigue, fluid retention, tinnitus, and headache may occur. Concurrent use of diuretics must be avoided, and patients should have a normal salt level in their diet.

Naproxen and the other NSAIDs should be used sparingly for patients over 50 years of age. However, even in young people, regular blood tests must be performed.

Fenoprofen (Nalfon)

For patients who cannot tolerate naproxen, or for whom it is ineffective, fenoprofen is one alternative. This drug carries an increased risk of nephrotoxicity, and renal function must be closely monitored. Fenoprofen is helpful for some patients with daily headache, and tiny doses have been used as a migraine prophylactic for children.

Dosage

Fenoprofen is always to be taken with food. The starting dose is one 600 mg pill per day, increasing to the usual migraine dose of one 600 mg pill two or three times per day. Doses of 200 mg per day may be given to children.

Side Effects

Very similar to naproxen in its side effects, fenoprofen, as mentioned, carries an increased risk of nephrotoxicity; kidney functions must be frequently assessed via blood tests.

Ketoprofen (Orudis)

Ketoprofen has proved helpful in preventing migraine, and is also useful for daily headaches in some patients.

Dosage

Starting dose is 75 mg once per day, taken with food. If this dosage does not control the headaches, and no GI side effects have occurred, the dose may be increased to 75 mg twice per day.

Side Effects

Side effects are similar to those of the other anti-inflammatories. Liver irritation is fairly common, so liver and kidney tests must be monitored regularly.

Flurbiprofen (Ansaid)

Flurbiprofen is a well tolerated NSAID with prostaglandin effects that render it very helpful for menstrual migraine (see Chapter 4).

Dosage

The usual dose is one pill (100 mg) twice a day, taken with food.

Side Effects

Side effects are similar to the other NSAIDs, and regular blood tests need to be performed.

Calcium Channel Blockers

Relatively new migraine preventives, the calcium blockers are very useful because of the absence of side effects. The weight gain or lethargy commonly seen with migraine preventives do not usually occur with calcium channel blockers. Constipation occurs frequently. The calcium blockers may not be as effective as antidepressants or beta blockers, but they generate less side effects. Verapamil is also helpful for cluster and chronic daily headache.

Verapamil (Isoptin, Calan, Veralan)

The most widely prescribed and most effective calcium blocker is verapamil, but it may take up to 6 weeks to become effective. The long acting slow release form (Isoptin SR or Calan SR), in 120, 180, and 240 mg tablets, is convenient for the patient. There is a generic slow release form available. Verapamil may be combined with any of the other first line medications. Raynaud's phenomenon is common among migraineurs, and verapamil is helpful for this as well as for preventing migraines.

Dosage

The initial dose, half of a 180 or 240 mg tablet, taken once per day, is quickly increased to 180 or 240 mg per day. Occasionally, it may be helpful to increase to 480 mg per day, checking for hypotension. The average dose is 180 to 240 mg per day. The 80 mg pills taken 3 or 4 times per day may be slightly more effective than the long acting preparation, but the once daily dosing of the long acting pills greatly increases compliance.

Side Effects

Many patients tolerate verapamil very well. However, constipation is very common. Allergic reactions (rashes), dizziness, insomnia, and anxiety are occasionally experienced. Occasionally, verapamil may cause or exacer-

TABLE 3.6. A Comparison of Side Effects among Calcium Blockers.

Side Effect	Nifedipine	Verapamil	Diltiazem
Constipation	Low	High	Low
Headache (muscle tension)	High	Medium	Medium
Hypotension	High	Medium	Medium
Fluid retention	Medium	Medium	Medium
AV-block	Low	Medium to high	Medium

bate existing chronic daily headaches. Fatigue is less common than with the beta blockers, but occurs at times. Peripheral edema may become a problem.

Miscellaneous Calcium Blockers (See Table 3.6)

Verapamil is the only calcium blocker available in the United States that has proven to be effective for migraine. Nifedipine (Procardia) has been used, and is occasionally helpful for migraine or cluster patients. The usual dose is 10 or 20 mg two to three times per day, or the Procardia XL (long acting) may be utilized. Procardia has a similar side effect profile as is seen with verapamil. Similarly, diltiazen (Cardizem) is occasionally prescribed for migraine patients, but verapamil is consistently more effective. Flunarizine is effective but is not available in the U.S.

Second Line Preventive Medication

Polypharmacy: Using Two First Line Medications Together

When first line preventives are ineffective, one option is to utilize two of them in combination. In general, polypharmacy is avoided, but when necessary, a combination of preventives is more effective than one drug alone. Dosages and side effects may be the same as for the medications individually.

Amitriptyline and Propranolol

Amitriptyline is often combined with propranolol, particularly when tachycardia induced by amitriptyline must be offset by a beta blocker. This combination is the one most commonly used for patients with "mixed" headaches (migraine along with chronic daily headaches).

NSAIDs with Other First Line Preventives

NSAIDs may be combined with any other first line preventives. Naproxen is often given with amitriptyline, propranolol, or verapamil as both a preventive and an abortive medication. When NSAIDs are combined with amitriptyline on a daily basis, liver functions need to be assessed.

TABLE 3.7. Quick Reference Guide: Second Line Migraine Preventive Therapy.

1. Polypharmacy: Two first line medications are used together. The combination of two preventives is more effective than one drug alone. Amitriptyline is often combined with propranolol, particularly if the tachycardia of the amitriptyline needs to be offset by a beta blocker. This combination is the most commonly used one for "mixed" headaches (migraine plus chronic daily headache). The NSAIDs may be combined with any of the other first line preventives. Thus, naproxen is often given with amitriptyline, propranolol, or verapamil. Naproxen or other NSAIDs are employed simultaneously as preventive and abortive medication.
2. Methysergide (Sansert): Extremely effective, but with more side effects than the other first line medications. Nausea, leg cramps, and dizziness are common. Screening for the very rare fibrosis must be done, and the drug should be stopped for 1 month every 5 or 6 months. Dosage is one to four pills per day, with food; try to attain the least possible dose.
3. Valproate (Depakote): This seizure medication is becoming increasingly popular for migraine prevention. Liver functions need to be monitored in the beginning of treatment. Side effects include lethargy, GI upset, depression, memory difficulties, weight gain, and alopecia. Dosage ranges from 250 to 2,000 mg per day, in divided doses. The average dose is 1,000 mg per day. Levels need to be checked for toxicity on the higher doses.

Propranolol and Verapamil

Propranolol and verapamil may cautiously be combined. Cardiac status, as well as blood pressure, needs to be checked. Small doses of each medication are usually used, such as propranolol LA 60 mg plus verapamil SR 180 mg. Other beta blockers may be combined with verapamil.

Miscellaneous Second Line Medications
Methysergide (Sansert)

An extremely effective migraine preventive, Sansert has declined in popularity because of the possible side effect of fibrosis. With judicious use, however, it can be relatively safe and effective. The goal is to use low doses (1 to 3 pills per day), and to stop the medication for a 1 month drug holiday every 5 to 6 months. If patients are advised of the frequent side effects that may occur when first starting Sansert, their compliance will be greatly enhanced. Because of the vasoconstriction, Sansert is more useful in younger age ranges, and after age 45 or 50, I attempt to avoid the use of Sansert. For certain patients, Sansert is the only effective medication.

Dosage

Sansert must be started at one pill or even one-half pill each day. The only pill available is 2 mg, and they are difficult to cut in half. The average dose is one pill taken twice a day, usually with food. Although five to six pills per day are occasionally more effective, Sansert is best limited to four pills per day.

TABLE 3.8. Prevention Medication: When to Proceed Very Quickly, with Two Medications at One Time.

1. With most patients we utilize one prevention medication at a time, in low doses, slowly raising the dose as needed. The patients appreciate this approach, and are prepared to wait for the medication to work, and are willing to switch medications, if necessary.
2. At times, patients may have become extremely frustrated with the headaches, and desire fast results. When the patients have moderate or severe chronic daily headaches, with bothersome migraines, it is justified to push ahead at a faster rate with a preventive approach. For instance, Elavil and verapamil, or Elavil and propranolol, may be instituted at the same time. Alternatively, doses may be pushed much faster than is usually done. The IV DHE repetitive protocol may be utilized, and at the same time, one or two preventive medications initiated. The amount of preventive medication utilized in the beginning depends upon the severity of the headaches and the frustration level of the patient.
3. Patients with new onset of severe headaches, usually daily headaches plus migraine, are often extremely upset and frustrated with the pain. In this situation, pushing preventive medication at a faster pace is justified.

Side Effects

Nausea is common, as is a hot feeling in the head and leg cramps. Some patients simply complain of "feeling weird." These reactions can be severe, so patients must be warned not to panic should the extreme side effects occur. Fibrosis has been reported, primarily when large doses are given over extended periods of time. Therefore, we use small doses with at least 1 month drug holiday every 5 to 6 months. This drug holiday is controversial, because it has not been proven to prevent fibrosis, and it may, at times, render the drug ineffective after restarting. During the drug holiday, a substitute may be employed in the form of small amounts of cortisone or another first line preventive. Alternatively, the Sansert may simply be stopped and the patient's headache pattern observed. If the patient remains improved, the Sansert is not restarted. With continued use of Sansert, frequent physical exams, blood and urine checks, and a once-per-year chest x-ray must be performed. Echocardiography of the heart, to assess for valvular dysfunction, should be part of the routine screening done while on Sansert. An MRI of the retroperitoneal space should be taken for fibrosis once per year. When fibrosis occurs, it usually reverses on cessation of Sansert. The actual incidence of fibrosis is very low, approximately one case out of 700 to 1,500 patients on Sansert for long periods of time. Because of the peripheral vasoconstriction, patients with coronary artery disease, previous thrombophlebitis, or any peripheral vascular disorders should not be placed on Sansert. Patients with hypertension should be monitored very closely while on Sansert. I do not usually use Sansert after age 45 to 50. With close monitoring, it is justified in occasional patients to utilize continuous Sansert without a drug holiday.

Valproate (Depakote)

This seizure medicine has been excellent for migraine, tension, and cluster headaches. Depakote may cause a mild hepatic irritation, but severe hepatotoxicity has only been observed in children who are usually on other seizure medications. There have been no cases of hepatic fatalities in patients over 10 years of age receiving Depakote as monotherapy. Depakote should be considered if the first line migraine preventives have failed, alone or in combination. Depakote is very helpful for chronic daily headache. Since we are using Depakote only as a second line therapy, when the first line drugs have not been effective, the rate of success will be lower in this group of refractive patients.

Dosage

Depakote is started with a low dose, one 250 mg tablet per day with food. The Depakote is a coated tablet. This dosage can be rapidly increased over 2 weeks to 1,000 mg per day (one 500 mg tablet twice a day). Side effects may limit increasing the dosage, and many patients continue at only 500 mg per day. Valproate blood levels should be drawn on doses of 1,000 mg per day or higher. The levels are drawn primarily to check for toxicity. Whether efficacy correlates with higher levels is not known. Depakote levels are usually higher during monotherapy than with poly-therapy. The effective dose of Depakote varies widely from patient to patient, with some patients requiring only 250 mg, and others needing 2,500 mg per day.

Side Effects

Nausea, gastritis, and sedation are frequently seen with Depakote. Weight gain occurs in almost one out of five patients, and is due to an increase in appetite. The weight gain is dose-related, and low doses are unlikely to produce an increase in weight. Depakote mildly impairs cognitive function in some patients. Hair loss occurs in about 5% of patients and is usually transient. Reduction in dose helps the alopecia, but the Depakote needs to be discontinued if alopecia continues unabated. Zinc may possibly be helpful for the alopecia. Hyperammonemia may occur and at times is associated with lethargy. A reduction in dose or discontinuation of Depakote is not usually necessary with hyperammonemia. Hepatotoxicity with liver failure is very rare, with no reported fatalities in patients above the age of 10 receiving valproate as monotherapy. The major risk for fatal hepatotoxicity is in the 0 to 2-year-old age range. A dose-related, reversible, and usually transient elevation in SGOT and SGPT occurs in up to 44% of patients. These liver enzymes usually decrease back to normal with time or with a reduction in dosage. Do not use valproate in patients with preexisting liver disease.

TABLE 3.9. Quick Reference Guide: Third Line Migraine Prevention.

1. Phenelzine (Nardil): This MAOI inhibitor (MAOI) is a powerful migraine and daily headache preventive medication. Phenelzine may be used alone, or in combination with amitriptyline, verapamil, or propranolol. Phenelzine is very helpful for depression, anxiety, and panic attacks. The risk of a hypertensive crisis is small but is a major drawback to the MAOIs. Dietary restrictions render MAOIs difficult for the patient. Side effects include insomnia and weight gain, both of which are often major problems. Dry mouth, fatigue, constipation, and cognitive effects may also occur. Patients need to be aware of the symptoms of hypertensive reactions. The usual dose is 45 mg each night (3 of the 15 mg tablets). This is adjusted up or down, and the range varies from one to five tablets per day.
2. Repetitive IV DHE therapy: Helpful for patients with frequent migraine, severe daily headache, status migraine, and cluster headache. Weeks of headache improvement is often seen. IV DHE is useful in patients withdrawing from analgesics. The protocol can be done in the office or hospital. In the office, the protocol consists of metoclopramide, 5 or 10 mg, and 2 Tums, followed in $\frac{1}{2}$ hour by the DHE. For the first dose, $\frac{1}{2}$ mg is given, and if it is well tolerated the subsequent doses are 1 mg. Three or four doses are given in the office, and up to nine in the hospital. Side effects include nausea, heat flashes, muscle contraction headache, leg cramps, diarrhea, and GI pain. The IV DHE is usually well tolerated and effective. After the DHE, patients are continued on prevention medication.
3. Amphetamines (Dextroamphetamine, Methamphetamine): Occasionally useful as a "last resort" therapy.

Salicylates should be limited, if possible, with valproate. A fine tremor that resembles essential tremor may appear with Depakote. This is dose-related and responds to either a reduction in dose or to propranolol. Mood swings and fatigue may occur, and may prompt discontinuation of Depakote. Depakote is strongly worth considering in refractory headache patients.

Third Line Migraine Preventive Medication

The third line approaches for migraine prophylaxis are: (1) MAO inhibitors; (2) MAO inhibitor plus a first line preventive; (3) intravenous DHE and (4) Amphetamines. These third line therapies are not instituted without first attempting other, less problematic, options.

MAO Inhibitors

The use of MAOIs, such as phenelzine, poses potentially serious problems. However, they can be helpful in severe, refractory migraine, and are very effective when utilized for chronic daily headache. Their strong antianxiety and antipanic effects are useful for many patients, as are the beneficial effects on depression. Patients must be selected carefully since they need to be vigilant about what they eat, and they cannot take OTC cold remedies. Given these restrictions, reponsible patients can use the

TABLE 3.10. Foods to Avoid while on Nardil.

Red wine or sherry, ale, and beer
Tenderized meats, caviar, dried or salted fish, herring, liver, fermented meats (pepperoni, summer sausage, salami, bologna)
Excessive caffeine, chocolate
Aged cheeses (only Velveeta is OK to eat)
Yogurt
Sour cream
Bananas, figs that are overripe, avocados
Yeast extracts
Soy sauce
Raisins
Fava beans

MAOIs with relative safety. The hypertensive crisis due to interactions with foods or drugs is a rare occurrence. (See Table 3.10) The MAOIs may be carefully combined with certain tricyclics, beta blockers, and calcium blockers. Sumatriptan cannot be used with the MAOIs. For any of the following medications, patients need to be informed of the side effects, as listed in the PDR and package insert.

Phenelzine (Nardil)

Nardil is the MAOI most frequently used for headache prevention. Nardil is often effective for refractive migraine, and is helpful for chronic daily headache. Nardil also relieves anxiety and depression.

Dosage

Beginning with one 15 mg tablet each night, the dose may be increased over 1 week to three tablets each night. By taking the medication only at night, interactions are much less likely to occur with tyramine foods. The usual dosage is 45 mg (3 tablets) each night. Some patients do well on 15 or 30 mg nightly, and others require 75 mg. Minimal doses lessen the likelihood of side effects. If 75 mg (5 pills) do not help, another medication should be employed and Nardil discontinued.

Side Effects

Side effects tend to be similar to those of the tricyclic antidepressants: dry mouth, constipation, insomnia, and weight gain. Tachycardia may occur. The major problems with Nardil are insomnia and weight gain. Switching to early morning dosing may help the insomnia. Agitation or other mood altering side effects may occur. Nardil is a very effective antidepressant and antianxiety drug. Hypotension may be a problem, and patients must have blood pressures checked both lying and standing (orthostatic). In very rare situations, where only Nardil has helped the patient but hypotension is a major problem, the hypotension may be counteracted by adding Florinef. Sedation can occur but is uncommon. Liver functions must be monitored via blood tests.

If water retention becomes a problem, careful use of diuretics may be helpful. Although it is not generally advisable to treat side effects of one medication with another medication, in situations where Nardil is the patient's only effective therapy for headache, we may have no other option but to treat the side effects. The most serious adverse effect, the hypertensive crisis, is uncommon, but may occur with the ingestion of certain foods. Meperidine (Demerol) or decongestants may not be used with MAO inhibitors. Patients should contact their physician prior to taking other drugs or OTC preparations. Excessive amounts of caffeine should be avoided.

To counteract the hypertensive crisis, should it occur, patients should carry capsules of Procardia, 20 mg. They would bite or cut the capsule and put it under the tongue for the following circumstances: a headache that is much different than their usual one, nausea and vomiting, dilated pupils, palpitations, neck or occipital pain that is different than their usual headache, diaphoresis with either cold, wet extremities or with a fever. They then must go to the emergency room for a blood pressure check. Among reliable headache patients, this crisis occurs very rarely.

Phenelzine Plus Verapamil

This very powerful combination for severe, refractive migraines must be monitored since hypotension is a problem. The usual dosage is two to four phenelzine pills (15 mg each) plus 120 to 240 mg of verapamil per day. Verapamil SR tablets are available in 120, 180, and 240 mg, allowing convenient once per day dosing. In addition to easing the migraines, verapamil minimizes the possibility of a hypertensive crisis. The dosages of both the phenelzine and the verapamil must be very slowly increased over 2 weeks, with frequent blood pressure checks. The usual precautions observed with the use of MAOIs must also be observed with this combination.

Phenelzine Plus Amitriptyline

This powerful combination of drugs for migraine, chronic daily headache, and depression is actually much less of a problem than was previously thought. Some evidence exists that the amitriptyline decreases the risk of a hypertensive crisis with the phenelzine. This combination is particularly helpful in cases where phenelzine is effective for the headaches but causes a severe sleep disorder. The same cautions must be followed with this combination as with phenelzine alone, but with this combination hypotension is more likely to occur than the hypertensive crisis, and blood pressure must be closely watched.

The usual dosage of phenelzine is two to four pills (15 mg per pill) per day, and 10 to 50 mg of amitriptyline per night.

Repetitive IV DHE

For patients with severe, frequent migraines or severe chronic daily headaches, repetitive IV DHE therapy has been very successful. Although usually performed in the hospital over 3 days, giving nine doses of DHE, the procedure may be done in the office without difficulty. Outpatient DHE allows this treatment to be available for those patients who do not wish to be hospitalized. IV DHE has proven very safe; serious side effects are rare, with only a few reported cases of claudication (that was reversible) and angina. The pharmacology of DHE is different than that of the other ergot preparations. It does not greatly constrict arteries, but is primarily a venoconstrictor. Serotonergic effects are most likely the mechanism of action. Although DHE is relatively safe for patients over the age of 50, caution must be used and lower doses given to those in older age ranges. Patients with peripheral vascular disease or heart disease must not be given DHE. DHE should be used with caution in patients with hypertension.

For the majority of patients, IV DHE has been successful in decreasing the intensity and frequency of headaches for a period of time. I have found that the effects of a course of DHE therapy usually last 1 or 2 months, with an occasional 6 or 8 month hiatus in the headaches. It is extremely effective for halting an acute migraine, as well as for preventing migraine attacks.

Side Effects

The usual side effects are nausea, a hot feeling in the head, tightness in the throat or chest, leg and muscle cramps, and a transient rise in blood pressure. Because of the nausea, which is common, an antiemetic pill or injection is given half an hour prior to the DHE. The tightness in the throat or chest rapidly stops and does not present a serious problem, for it is of muscular or GI origin. An EKG should be done if this occurs. A transient muscle tension headache may ensue following the DHE, and diarrhea is occasionally a problem.

Office Protocol for IV DHE

The office protocol is as follows: give Reglan, one-half or one 10 mg pill, with several Tums. One-half hour later, slowly give $\frac{1}{2}$ mg IV DHE. If well tolerated, give another $\frac{1}{2}$ mg, for a total of 1 cc as the first dose. I do not usually utilize a hep-lock. If the first dose is well tolerated, as it usually is, the entire 1 mg of DHE can be given at the next treatment. Patients may take the Reglan pill at home, prior to arriving for the DHE. Reglan is not usually very sedating, so that patients can drive, which is a tremendous advantage. The patient must be alert prior to driving after the DHE. If nausea is a problem, the dose is either lowered to $\frac{1}{2}$ or $\frac{3}{4}$ mg, or stronger antiemetic medications are utilized. Phenergan, 25 mg PO or IM, may be utilized. Alternatively, Vistaril, 25 mg PO or IM, may be effective and is less sedating than Phenergan. Compazine, 10 to 25 mg PO or 5 mg IM, is a very effective antiemetic. Compazine may induce severe side effects (agitation or extrapyramidal reactions). Thorazine is a very effective medication to combat nausea, but with an increased incidence of side effects. Most patients are able to tolerate DHE with the Reglan as an antiemetic.

Blood pressure and pulse must be monitored before and after the DHE is given, and it is not unusual for the blood pressure to rise slightly after the DHE.

The office protocol is usually performed twice per day for 2 or 3 days, or a total of four to six doses.

Hospital Protocol for IV DHE

In the hospital, more doses may be administered in 1 day than in the office. We attempt to give a total of nine doses of DHE. The protocol is the same as in the office, beginning with only one pill of Reglan and, if necessary, progressing to stronger antiemetic medications. The goal is to utilize doses of DHE that are subnauseating. Detoxification from analgesics is somewhat easier in the hospital than as an outpatient. If needed, IV fluids may be given in the hospital. However, the overwhelming majority of patients greatly appreciate receiving DHE as outpatients.

In the hospital, doses of DHE are given at 8 hour intervals. If nausea is extreme and the other nausea medications have proved ineffective, Thorazine, 25 to 50 mg IM, is administered prior to the DHE. Alternatively, Reglan or Compazine may be given intravenously for severe nausea. IV DHE is extremely effective for a variety of headache types, including migraine, tension, and cluster.

Amphetamines

As a "last resort," patients may experience less migraine or CDH with Methylphenidate, Dexedrine, or Desoxyn. Insomnia, anxiety, and dependance are possible problems. Doses should be minimized. Doses of Methylphenidate vary from 20 mg to 40 mg per day. Dexedrine is usually dosed at 5 mg or 10 mg BID. Desoxyn is dosed at 2.5 mg or 5 mg BID. Side effects, as listed in the PDR, need to be explained to the patient.

CHAPTER 4

Hormones and Headaches

Introduction

In women migraineurs, the female sex hormones, progestins and estrogens, exert a profound influence on the number and severity of migraine headaches. Why this occurs, and the mechanisms involved, remains unclear. Menstrual migraines generate an enormous amount of suffering because they tend to be more severe than nonmenstrually related headaches. In addition, they are often resistant to the usual migraine medication strategies. Headaches often decline in severity during pregnancy, but when present they are difficult to treat, because of the limited number of safe medications available. During menopause, headaches may follow any pattern, and they often improve after this time. When women require hormone replacement therapy, there are certain hormonal approaches that may help limit the headaches. Oral contraceptives may induce or exacerbate headache, or, less often, the headaches may improve. The majority of the time, the birth control pill does not influence migraine; however, it is important to be aware of the possibility of migraine exacerbation with the oral contraceptives.

Menstrual Migraine

Menstrually related migraine occurs prior, during, or after menstruation. Many women with menstrual migraine also experience an exacerbation with ovulation. Most often, the woman will also experience migraines that occur at other times of the cycle that are not hormonally influenced. Occasionally, women may suffer menstrual migraine alone, without other headaches.

In several studies, progestin and estrogen levels have been found to be increased premenstrually in women migraineurs. However, others have not discovered this difference. Luteinizing hormone (LH) and follicle-stimulating hormone (FSH) levels, as well as testosterone levels, have been the same in migraineurs as in controls. Estrogen withdrawal may produce migraine headaches, but the exact mechanism of this is uncertain.

Estrogen and progesterone influence serotonin receptors. Estrogen withdrawal exerts a profound effect on hypothalamic control machanisms. Prostaglandins have been found in increased concentrations in women experiencing menstrual migraine.

Prostaglandin synthesis is blocked by the NSAIDs, which may help to explain the role of the NSAIDs in treating menstrual migraine. Opioid peptide levels may be altered during menstrual migraine. All of the above factors may play a role in menstrual migraine. For any of the following medications, patients need to be informed of the side effects, as listed in the PDR and package insert.

Treatment of Menstrual Migraine

Menstrual migraine is often severe, refractory, and prolonged. However, many women suffer only a mild or moderate 1 day migraine, easily managed with the first line abortive migraine medications (see Chapter 2), such as Excedrin or ibuprofen. At times, the standard migraine preventive medications help the menstrual migraines, such as propranolol or amitriptyline. For those women who experience severe, prolonged menstrual migraines, the preventive approaches include the following: (1)

TABLE 4.1. Quick Reference Guide: Treatment of Menstrual Migraine.

Abortive Treatment

The abortive therapy follows the general abortive therapy for migraine (see Chapter 2). Cortisone (Prednisone, Decadron) is very effective for many women; it is utilized in very limited amounts. Women may self-administer IM DHE, sumatriptan, or ketorolac (Toradol). The severe intensity of menstrual migraines often dictates stronger abortive measures.

Preventive Treatment

1. NSAIDs (Naproxen, etc.): Effective for many women, and usually well tolerated. These are started 3 days prior to the expected onset of the headache. Many NSAIDs have been utilized, including naproxen, ibuprofen, flurbiprofen, meclofenamate sodium, etc. GI upset is common.
2. Ergotamine derivatives: The usual forms of ergots utilized include: ergotamine tartrate, Bellergal-S, ergonovine, DHE, and methysergide. These are started 1 to 3 days prior to the expected onset of the headache. Ergots are poorly tolerated, with frequent GI upset and nausea. Ergotamine rebound may occur, but is unusual when ergots are used for menstrual migraine.
3. Hormonal approaches: Tamoxifen (Nolvadex) competes with estrogen, and is utilized for 7 to 14 days. Five to 10 mg per day is the usual dose. Usually well tolerated, but recent reports (from laboratory animal studies) of liver CA have appeared. Synthetic estrogen preparations (ethinyl estradiol or micronized estradiol) are sometimes effective. Side effects are common. Estrogen plus methyltestosterone may be the most effective menstrual migraine prophylactic regimen. Side effects are many, but the dose for menstrual migraine is small. Danazol (Danocrine) is a synthetic androgen occasionally effective for menstrual migraine. There are many side effects that limit the use of this drug.

NSAIDs, such as naproxen (Naprosyn, Anaprox), ibuprofen (Motrin), or flurbiprofen (Ansaid); (2) ergotamine (Cafergot, Ergostat) or ergot derivatives, such as Bellergal-S, ergonovine, DHE, and methysergide (Sansert); and (3) hormonal approaches, such as tamoxifen (Nolvadex), estrogen, estrogen plus androgen, or danazol (Danocrine).

Abortive Treatment

Abortive treatment of menstrual migraine usually follows the abortive therapy of migraine, as outlined in Chapter 2. For severe menstrual migraines, cortisone is one of the more effective treatments, usually Decadron or prednisone. These are discussed in Chapter 2. Decadron, 4 mg tablets, or prednisone, 20 mg pills, are usually limited to four pills per month at most, and are taken every 6 hours, as needed. Other stronger abortive measures include IM ketorolac (Toradol), or IM DHE, both of which the patient may self-administer. If these strategies fail, at times a strong narcotic, such as meperidine (Demerol) with a powerful antiemetic, such as chlorpromazine (Thorazine), helps to avoid emergency room visits. The intense severity of menstrual migraines necessitates stronger abortive measures in many women. These abortive migraine strategies are discussed extensively in Chapter 2.

Preventive Medications

Nonsteroidal Anti-inflammatories

The anti-inflammatories remain the mainstay of menstrual migraine preventive therapy, not because they are extremely effective, but because the side effects are less than with the other medications that are used. The anti-inflammatory is usually begun 3 days prior to the expected onset of the headache; if the patient experiences migraine beginning on the first day of the period, the NSAID is instituted 3 days prior to the expected onset of menses. The medication is continued for several days past the point of the "expected" headache. When the menstrual periods are irregular, medication is usually started the first day of the period, or when the woman feels that the menses is about to begin. Women who tend to experience the headache prior to, during, or after the menses require a much longer period of preventive therapy than women with premenstrual migraines. The timing of preventive therapy for hormonal headaches is often extremely difficult.

Naproxen (Naprosyn, Anaprox) has been the most widely studied medication for prevention of menstrual migraine. For a complete discussion of naproxen for headache, please see Chapters 2 and 3. The usual dose is one Naprosyn 500 mg pill, or one Anaprox D.S. 550 mg pill, taken with food each day. This may be increased to one tablet twice per day. GI side effects are common, but otherwise the naproxen is well tolerated. Fluid retention may occur. The naproxen may also be utilized as an abortive agent once the headache begins.

Ibuprofen (Motrin) is available over the counter, and is well tolerated. It is also very effective for many women's menstrual cramps. The effective dose of ibuprofen varies widely, from as little as 400 mg per day to 2,400 mg per day, in divided doses. As with naproxen, GI side effects are common. Ibuprofen may also be used as an abortive medication. Ibuprofen is also discussed in Chapter 2.

Flurbiprofen (Ansaid) is an effective and generally well tolerated anti-inflammatory. The usual dose is one 100 mg pill twice per day, or, if tolerated, the 2 tablets may be taken at the same time. GI side effects are common, as with any anti-inflammatory. Flurbiprofen may be used abortively.

Many other NSAIDs have been utilized for menstrual migraine prophylaxis. These include ketoprofen (Orudis), meclofenamate sodium (Meclomen), mefenamic acid (Ponstel), and fenoprofen (Nalfon). These are all probably as effective as naproxen or flurbiprofen. Some women will tolerate or respond to one anti-inflammatory significantly better than to another. It is sometimes worthwhile to attempt treatment with several anti-inflammatories as preventive medications prior to abandoning this class.

Ergotamine Derivatives

Ergotamine may be utilized for the prevention of menstrual migraine, with minimal risk for developing ergotamine rebound headaches. Ergotamine may also be used abortively for the acute headache. The forms of ergots that are employed are: (1) ergotamine tartrate, (2) Bellergal-S, (3) ergonovine, (4) DHE, and (5) methysergide (Sansert).

Ergotamine Tartrate

Although ergotamine is usually considered to be a migraine abortive, it is occasionally helpful as a preventive for certain forms of migraine or cluster headache. Ergostat sublingual pills are "pure" ergotamine tablets, to be taken sublingually or swallowed. Each tablet contains 2 mg of ergotamine tartrate. One tablet should be swallowed each day, beginning one day prior to the expected onset of the migraine, and continued until the headache period has passed. If the woman usually experiences a migraine on the first day of the period, the ergostat would be started 1 day earlier, and used for 3 or 4 days. The possibility of rebound headaches needs to be considered when utilizing ergots in this preventive fashion. Cafergot tablets or suppositories may be used in this manner as preventives, but the Cafergot adds caffeine to the ergotamine. One or two Cafergot tablets, or one suppository, would be used one day prior to the expected headache, and continued until the "danger" period for the headaches has elapsed.

Frequent side effects of ergots are nausea or severe GI upset, nervousness, and leg cramps. Besides these common effects, the possibility always exists that daily use of these may actually exacerbate migraine headaches; they need to be discontinued if this occurs. The ergots are discussed extensively in Chapter 2.

Bellergal-S

Bellergal-S contains 40 mg of phenobarbital, 0.6 mg of ergotamine tartrate and tartrazine, and 0.2 mg of l-alkaloids of belladonna. The phenobarbital is sedating, and this may be useful for perimenstrual insomnia. The 0.6 mg of ergotamine is less than the 1 mg in a Cafergot tablet, but this is enough to prevent migraine in some patients. The usual dose is one tablet each night, beginning one night prior to the expected onset of the headache. This may be increased to one tablet twice per day, or two tablets each night. The Bellergal-S is then continued for several days past the "danger" period for the headache. Sedation may occur secondary to the phenobarbital, and the usual side effects of ergots may also be present, such as GI upset and nausea.

Ergonovine

Ergonovine is generally a well tolerated ergotamine derivative. Ergonovine is occasionally effective for both cluster and migraine. Ergotrate is the brand name that is available, but is often available in pharmacies in only very limited quantities. Compounding pharmacists are easily able to formulate ergonovine from the powder in any desired strength. The primary use for ergonovine in medicine is to increase the frequency, duration, and strength of uterine contractions, thus treating and preventing postabortal and postpartum uterine hemorrhage.

The Ergotrate brand is available as 0.2 mg tablets, and the usual dose is 0.2 mg 2 to 4 times per day. This would be started 1 day prior to the expected onset of the headache, and continued for 2 or 3 days after the headache period. Side effects are usually somewhat less than with the standard ergotamines, but nausea and GI upset are common. Leg cramps or anxiety also may occur, but are generally encountered less often than with other ergotamines.

DHE

DHE is primarily an abortive medication, but occasionally it is useful for the prevention of menstrual migraine. The only commercially available form is the IM injection, but nasal spray or suppositories may be formulated. DHE is also formulated as an oral capsule, but the absorption is very poor. For menstrual migraine prophylaxis, DHE is given as a 1 mg injection once a day, beginning 1 day prior to the expected onset of the headache and continued for 1 day after the headache period. Alternatively, two nasal sprays may be used each day during the same period, or one 2 mg DHE suppository. Intravenous DHE is effective for menstrual migraine prophylaxis, but is not very practical for regular monthly use.

The usual side effects of DHE are nausea, throat or chest tightness, mild muscle contraction headache, leg cramps, and a "hot" feeling about the head. DHE is usually very well tolerated, and may be used during the menstrual time as both a preventive and abortive medication. DHE is discussed extensively in Chapters 2 and 3.

Methysergide (Sansert)

This powerful migraine preventive medication may be utilized perimenstrually for the prevention of menstrual migraines. The 2 mg tablets, one each day with food, are initiated 1 day prior to the expected onset of the headache, and continued for 2 or 3 days past the headache period. If tolerated, the dose may be pushed to 2 or 3 tablets each day, in divided doses. The side effects are often severe, with a high incidence of severe GI upset, nausea, and leg cramps. In addition, many patients experience a flushed and hot feeling about the head. Dizziness or lightheadedness may be extreme. Patients need to be warned about the possibility of these side effects, and informed that they will usually stop in a matter of hours. When tolerated, methysergide is often a very helpful migraine preventive medication. Methysergide is also discussed in Chapter 3.

Hormonal Approaches to Menstrual Migraine Prevention

If the above therapies have not been effective and the menstrual migraines are very severe and debilitating, it is justified to consider stronger approaches, such as the use of hormonal therapy. Prior to utilizing hormonal therapies, women need to be informed of associated risks, as listed in a major drug reference guide.

Tamoxifen (Nolvadex)

Tamoxifen competes with estrogen in target tissues, and is primarily used as an adjuvant breast cancer therapy. Gynecomastia and mastalgia have also been treated with tamoxifen. In low doses, I use tamoxifen for the prevention of menstrual migraine. Tamoxifen is one of the more effective menstrual migraine prevention medications. In some women, tamoxifen has decreased migraines and daily headaches at other times of the month as well.

Tamoxifen is available as a 10 mg pill. The usual dose is 10 mg per day for 7 to 14 days, usually given just prior to the menstrual period. Starting the tamoxifen earlier in the cycle, such as 1 week after menses, may be more effective in some women. The dose may be lowered to 5 mg, or increased to 15 or 20 mg per day. The usual dose for the treatment or prevention of breast cancer is 10 or 20 mg per day, but this has been increased in some patients.

Adverse effects are usually absent or mild, and include nausea, hot flashes, and menstrual irregularities. Rashes, vaginal bleeding, and vaginal discharges may occur. Other side effects such as leukopenia, weight gain, edema, headache, shortness of breath, loss of appetite, pain in the legs, blurred vision, and dizziness may occur but are rare with the low doses utilized for headache. Malignant liver tumors have been reported in animal studies; however, the animal studies have, in general, been conducted with very large doses. The patient needs to be informed of the association of liver carcinomas, at least in laboratory studies, and the use of tamoxifen. Uterine CA has also been reported.

Estrogen

During the normal menstrual cycle, there is a decrease in levels of estrogen during the late luteal phase. This may be a prominent factor in triggering the headache. Estrogen alleviates the headache in some women and exacerbates the headache in others. Progesterone is generally not effective for menstrual migraine, and will often increase headaches. Percutaneous estradiol gel, used perimenstrually, has been effective in the prevention of menstrual migraine, but this preparation is not available in the United States. I primarily use oral estrogen, usually ethinyl estradiol (Estinyl), 0.05 mg, or micronized estradiol (Estrace), 1 or 2 mg. Premarin, which is a natural conjugated estrogen, has an irregular absorption, and the fluctuating estrogen levels may contribute to headache. In addition, Premarin has miscellaneous natural compounds, equine-derived, that may possibly trigger headache. The synthetic estrogen preparations are, in theory, better for headache patients. The estradiol transdermal system (Estraderm) gives very consistent absorption of estrogen, and is useful for menstrual migraine prophylaxis. Since the use of estrogens is contraindicated during pregnancy, this issue needs to be explained prior to initiating therapy.

The usual dose of estrogen is 0.05 mg of ethinyl estradiol (Estinyl), one tablet each day for 5 days prior to menses; this may be continued for 2 days after the onset of menstrual flow. I will usually utilize estrogen for a 1 week period of time. Alternatively, Estrace may be used, usually 1 mg per day. The estrogen transdermal patch, Estraderm, may be utilized, with the 0.05 mg patches. The total estradiol content is 4 mg, and the release rate is 0.05 mg per 24 hours. The patch is changed twice weekly, and utilized for a total of 7 days. The idea is to minimize the length of time on estrogen, but to use the medication for a long enough time for it to be effective. The women who are placed on estrogens, or any hormonal therapy, have very severe, prolonged migraines. The debilitating nature of these severe menstrual migraines justifies the use of stronger medication approaches.

Side effects of estrogens are many, and include: breakthrough bleeding, dysmenorrhea, amenorrhea, menstrual flow changes, endometrial hyperplasia, vaginal candidiasis, nausea, abdominal cramps, colitis or cholestatic jaundice, alopecia or hives, hirsutism, headache, dizziness, depression, decrease or increase in weight, edema, decreased libido, tenderness of the breasts, and chloasma. Estrogens may also increase the risk of endometrial carcinoma. Breast cancer may be influenced by estrogens. Estrogens are contraindicated during pregnancy or with a history of thrombophlebitis or thromboembolic disorders. Preexisting uterine leiomyomas may grow during estrogen therapy. Although small doses are utilized for limited periods of time, women on estrogens should be followed closely by their gynecologist.

Estrogen plus Methyltestosterone

The addition of small amounts of methyltestosterone may enhance the efficacy of the estrogen regime for menstrual migraine prophylaxis. Methyltestosterone is a synthetic derivative of testosterone, with anabolic and, to a lesser degree, androgenic properties. With the use of androgens, endogenous testosterone release is inhibited via the feedback inhibition of LH. The doses utilized for menstrual migraine prophylaxis are small, and the drug is used for the 7 days that the estrogens are given. The standard indications for the use of androgens include hypogonadism, androgen deficiency, breast cancer, and postpartum breast pain and engorgement.

The typical dose is 5 mg of methyltestosterone each day. The tablets are usually only available in 10 and 25 mg sizes, and we use one half of a 10 mg tablet. The dose is given at the same time as the estrogen, usually for 7 days.

Side effects are many and include: amenorrhea or other menstrual problems, virilization, hirsutism, acne, edema, nausea, cholestatic jaundice, changes in libido, headache, nervousness, depression, excitation, insomnia, rash, and alterations in liver function tests. However, in the small doses utilized, for limited times, side effects are not common.

Danazol (Danocrine)

Danazol is a synthetic androgen that suppresses the pituitary-ovarian axis by decreasing output of gonadotropins by the pituitary. Danazol decreases the output of LH and FSH. The primary use of danazol is in the treatment of endometriosis. It is occasionally a useful agent in the therapy of menstrual migraine.

Several dosing regimens have been utilized with danazol. The short course of danazol involves treatment for 3 to 5 days prior to the expected onset of the headache, and for 2 to 3 days after. The longer course consists of danazol for 25 days on, and 5 days off. Although the utilization of danazol for a longer period of time may be more effective, the side effects are much more pronounced.

I usually utilize danazol for 3 to 5 days prior to the expected time of the headache, and for 3 days after. The dose is started at 200 mg once per day, and titrated up or down, usually utilizing doses of 100 to 300 mg per day. Danocrine is available as 50 and 200 mg capsules. Capsules render dosage adjustments more difficult than with tablets.

Adverse reactions are many, and include the following: acne, hirsutism, edema, sweating and flushing, nervousness, hepatic dysfunction, weight gain, deepening of the voice, decrease in breast size, vaginitis, emotional lability, rashes, headache, insomnia, fatigue, changes in libido, alopecia, and increased blood pressure. However, in the low doses for short periods of time that we utilize danazol for menstrual migraines, side effects tend to be mild.

Headache During Pregnancy

Migraine often diminishes during pregnancy. However, the headaches may at times be increased during the pregnancy, or the onset of migraine may occur during pregnancy. Organic causes for headache need to be considered and excluded in pregnant woman with severe headaches. Treatment of the migraine or CDH during pregnancy consists of utilization of the nonmedication techniques, such as ice and relaxation therapy, and judicious use of small amounts of medication. The abortive medications are predominantly used, with preventive therapy reserved for only the most resistant headaches. Although we attempt to maintain a drug free pregnancy, severe headaches require therapy, and if the physician does not adequately treat the headaches, most women will resort to OTC preparations. Women need to be informed of any risks to the fetus, as listed in the PDR or "Drug Facts and Comparisons".

Acetaminophen is the primary abortive medication utilized during pregnancy, and may be combined with small amounts of caffeine, such as in Aspirin Free Excedrin. Although acetaminophen is mild, combining it with caffeine, lying down in a dark room, and utilizing ice about the head may be all that is necessary. Meperidine (Demerol) is relatively safe during pregnancy, and may be used orally or formulated as a suppository by a compounding pharmacist. Acetaminophen with codeine is also relatively safe during pregnancy. These narcotics should be used in small amounts, usually limited to 15 or 20 tablets per month (meperidine, 50 mg, or codeine, $\frac{1}{2}$ grain). Antiemetics should be reserved only for severe nausea and vomiting, and then used in small amounts. I usually utilize the 25 mg suppositories of promethazine (Phenergan).

TABLE 4.2. Treatment of Headache During Pregnancy.

Limit, minimize medications.
Ice packs, relaxation therapy, diet.
Caffeine, acetaminophen prn.
If above not effective, utilize small amounts of analgesics such as codeine or meperidine.
   Meperidine may be formulated as a suppository by compounding pharmacists.
For frequent, severe, intractable headache, prophylactic medication may be utilized. Beta
   blockers, such as propranolol (Inderal), are most commonly used. These should be
   stopped during the last month of pregnancy. In addition, medication must be minimized
   during the first trimester.

Prophylactic medication is occasionally necessary during pregnancy, because the migraines are frequent and severe or the daily headaches are intolerable. I usually institute a beta blocker such as propranolol (Inderal), but metoprolol, nadolol, timolol, or atenolol may be used. The beta blocker should be discontinued 3 weeks prior to delivery. The lowest possible dose needs to be employed. During the first trimester, all medication should be avoided or minimized, if possible. At levels 5 to 50 times the maximum recommended doses in humans, embryotoxic effects of the beta blockers have been demonstrated in laboratory animals. Although teratogenicity has not been reported in humans, several problems may occur during delivery. These include neonatal apnea, bradycardia, low Apgar scores, hypoglycemia, hypothermia, oliguria, etc. Women need to be given complete information on any medication that they are given during pregnancy, as listed in major sources such as the PDR, and risks need to be completely discussed and understood.

When beta blockers are not effective or are contraindicated, I usually use amitriptyline if daily preventive medication is necessary. Very low doses, such as 10 or 25 mg, need to be employed. The patient should be fully informed of possible teratogenicity. Isolated reports of limb reduction abnormalities have been reported, and the safety of tricyclic compounds has not been established with use during pregnancy. When the headaches are severe, and the woman is fully informed, amitriptyline may, with caution, be utilized.

Headache During Menopause and Post-Hysterectomy

Migraine follows several different pathways during and after the menopause. The headaches often increase in frequency or severity, but at times they may cease altogether. Many women do not experience any change in the migraine pattern. After hysterectomy or oophorectomy, there is also no consistent pattern to the headaches. They may greatly improve after the surgery, but more often the migraines increase.

The confusion surrounding menopausal headaches is increased by the fact that some women improve with estrogen replacement therapy and others experience more headaches. In women placed on estrogens and cyclic progestins, a moderate or severe increase in migraine should initiate a change in the hormone regimen. At times, it is necessary to discontinue the hormones completely. In women who have not had a hysterectomy, cyclic progestins are necessary, and these are the primary culprit in the exacerbation of the headaches. In addition, the withdrawal of estrogen for a number of days may trigger migraine. In women who have undergone hysterectomy, continuous estrogen therapy for the entire month, without a break, is often the best approach for the headaches.

When choosing an estrogen preparation, the synthetic compounds seem to create less migraine than Premarin. The equine-derived conjugated estrogens (Premarin) are not absorbed at a steady rate, and contain many natural compounds that could possibly trigger headache. Ethinyl estradiol (Estinyl), micronized estradiol (Estrace), esterified estrogens (Estratab), and estropipate (Ogen) are commonly used oral preparations. Estraderm is a transdermal estradiol that delivers a consistent blood level of estrogen. Depo-Estradiol is estradiol cypionate that is injected once every month. Many women will experience less migraine with this once per month injection. The effect of estrogen dose on migraine varies, with some women improving with increased doses, and others experiencing more headaches.

Progestins are utilized primarily to prevent endometrial cancer, reduce the risk of breast cancer, increase new bone formation, and prevent osteoporosis. The progestins may exacerbate headache, however. It is helpful to keep the dose to a minimum, and to utilize the progestins for the minimum number of days. However, some women have fewer migraines when on continuous low dose progestins throughout the month.

The addition of androgens (methyltestosterone) may help to alleviate certain symptoms of the menopause. Women often have improved libido, increased feelings of well-being, decreased depression, and improvement in headaches while on androgens. Methyltestosterone is occasionally helpful for menstrual and menopausal migraine. The androgens are utilized along with the estrogen, on the same days. Combination preparations are available, such as Estratest tablets, which consists of methyltestosterone (2.5 mg), and esterified estrogens (1.25 mg). Injectable forms are also available. A typical regimen would include one tablet of Estratest from day 1 through 25, and a progestin added from day 13 through 25.

CHAPTER 5

Migraine Headache Sample Case Studies

Sample Case History: Severe Migraine with Mild Chronic Daily Headache

Julie is 20 years old with severe, prolonged 2 to 3 day migraines twice per month. She also has mild chronic tension headache (CDH). She has difficulty sleeping and is mildly anxious. She occasionally utilizes an inhaler for asthma.

With only two migraines per month and mild CDH, a case could be made against prevention medication. However, with the severity and length of Julie's migraines (4 to 6 total days of severe migraine per month), prophylactic medications are indicated. Amitriptyline (Elavil) would be a good choice because of the headaches, insomnia, and anxiety. The asthma limits our selection of medication. We start with amitriptyline, 10 mg per night, increasing after 5 days to 25 mg each night. It is very important with amitriptyline to begin with a tiny dose (10 mg) as many patients cannot tolerate more than 5 or 10 mg. If patients are very tired upon awakening, I instruct them to take the amitriptyline at 7 or 8 pm instead of prior to sleeping. As an abortive, I give Julie a choice of Midrin and/or Anaprox D.S., warning her that asthma may be worse with Anaprox. The abortive medications should not be taken for the mild daily headaches, as we try not to "chase" after daily headaches with pain medications. This avoids the rebound headache situation.

Julie calls 6 days later, and the daily headache is gone but she is very lethargic. We now back off on the amitriptyline from 25 mg back to 10 mg. One month later, the daily headaches are still improved, and the Midrin and Anaprox help the migraines, but the migraines continue to last 2 to 3 days. At this point, we could add more prevention medication (daily Anaprox, increased amitriptyline, or a calcium blocker), but, in general, we want to minimize medication. Thus, simply treating the migraines with stronger "as needed" medication is the best choice.

Julie is now given Cafergot, from which she becomes nervous and nauseated. The ergotamine sublingual pills (Ergostat) help somewhat, but the next day she has her severe headache back again. Julie does not wish to utilize an injection, but if she did, Imitrex (sumatriptan) would be a consideration. We then proceed to Decadron, 4 mg tablets, and instruct her to take one-half tablet every 4 to 6 hours with food for a severe headache that lasts more than 1 day. This is very often the most effective treatment for severe migraines, and it works for Julie. We need to limit the Decadron to two full pills, or 8 mg, per month at most.

Two months later, the daily headaches are back again, and we increase the amitriptyline from 10 to 25 mg per night. She is no longer fatigued on this dose. If she became fatigued, we would need to go back to 10 mg of amitriptyline and add protriptyline (Vivactil), 5 mg each morning, or switch completely off amitriptyline to nortriptyline (Pamelor). Protriptyline is not sedating and is effective for daily headaches, but not nearly as effective for migraines as is amitriptyline. Protriptyline never causes weight gain, but has severe anticholinergic effects. Nortriptyline is less sedating than amitriptyline, but much more expensive and not as effective. DHE, either by self-injection or by nasal inhaler, is another good possibility for her severe migraines. If she does not wish to try DHE, as many patients do not because of the cost and the need for an injection, a butalbital compound may be given. Esgic or Fioricet (these are the same) would be a good choice for Julie because they do not contain aspirin and she has asthma. However, among the butalbital compounds, Fiorinal, which has aspirin, is the most effective. Do not use the generic butalbital medications.

Sample Case History: Severe Chronic Daily Headache

John is a 28-year-old man with a 3 year history of severe daily headaches and a true migraine every 3 months. It is very unusual to find patients with daily headaches who do not also have occasional migraine headaches, whether they are once per week or every 3 months. John has taken Fiorinal in the past, which helped, but now takes six to eight Excedrin per day. He also drinks four cups of coffee a day. He does not sleep well.

In this situation, it is important to stop the Excedrin, as John is probably contributing to his headaches by overusing this medication. He most likely is experiencing, to some degree, rebound headaches. His Excedrin, with 65 mg (about one cup of coffee) of caffeine, and his coffee intake add up to a large amount of caffeine per day. This needs to be decreased to the equivalent of three cups of coffee per day or less. A preventive medication should be instituted, particularly one that may help his sleeping. Amitriptyline is always a good choice with which to start, 10 mg for the first 4 nights, and then increasing to 25 mg. Biofeedback or relaxation therapy should be suggested. He needs to be told not to "chase" after the headaches all day with pain medication, but to allow the prevention medications to work. John is given Anaprox D.S. to use on an "as needed" basis.

John calls 5 days later. He is very lightheaded and fatigued on amitriptyline. He has stopped the Excedrin, and is having severe withdrawal headaches. He needs to be urged not to retreat back to his Excedrin, which many patients will do. If patients are convinced that the analgesics, when overused, actually cause their headaches and inhibit the efficacy of the preventives, they are more likely to stop overusing the pain medications. John's sleeping is improved while off the Excedrin and on Amitriptyline. He states that the Anaprox does help to a small degree. At this point, the preventive medication needs to be changed to a milder tricyclic, such as nortriptyline (Pamelor), at a low dose (10 mg). The Pamelor may have the same side effects as amitriptyline, but he is more likely to tolerate this regimen. The Anaprox is continued as an "as needed" medication.

One week later, John calls stating that he would like Fiorinal to "get him through". He is advised to push the Pamelor to 20 mg at night for 3 nights, and then 30 mg per night. He is not having problems with the Pamelor, but it has not helped. Do not fall into the trap of giving Fiorinal in this daily headache situation, unless all other avenues have not worked. We do not prescribe any Fiorinal.

John comes in 2 weeks later; the severity of the daily headache is down to a moderate level, and he is sleeping better. The Anaprox does not help. At this point, if he is not tired, the Pamelor may be pushed to as high as 150 mg, but he is fatigued on the 30 mg doses of Pamelor. To attempt to improve his daily headaches at this point, a nonsedating antidepressant needs to be instituted, such as Prozac or Vivactil. The Pamelor is decreased to one 25 mg capsule each night. We add Vivactil, 5 mg, one-half pill each morning for 4 days, then increasing to one pill each morning. Vivactil frequently causes dry mouth and dizziness, but almost never causes weight gain, and fatigue is uncommon.

John comes into the office, where his pulse is 98 per minute, and his blood pressure is 138/90. The tricyclics, particularly the Vivactil, will often raise the pulse, and at times the blood pressure. His headaches are improved, but he remains with a mild to moderate daily headache. At this point, we have several choices, including adding a small amount of a beta blocker to lower the pulse and blood pressure, or simply leaving the medication alone. Beta blockers are very useful in combination with the tricyclics, as they help the headaches, and offset the tachycardia of the tricyclics. Hypotension may become a problem with this combination, however. Fluoxetine (Prozac) does have a major advantage over the older tricyclics in that it does not usually increase the pulse or blood pressure.

At this point, when deciding whether to add another medication, thereby increasing side effects, the patient's entire situation needs to be assessed. In John's situation, he had been addicted to Excedrin and he previously experienced very severe headaches. Because he remains with headaches that are moderate on a daily basis, it is justified to initiate a small amount of a beta blocker. Nadolol (Corgard) is added, one-half of a 40 mg tablet for 4 days, then increasing to the whole 40 mg tablet. Corgard is particularly easy to work with because the scored tablets allow for easy dosage adjustments. He is now on small amounts of three medications; 30 mg of Pamelor, 5 mg of Vivactil, and 40 mg of Corgard. If we drop the Pamelor, he will probably have more headaches and he will not sleep as well. At this point, we would just leave the medication alone if the headaches are sufficiently improved. We will not retreat back to daily painkillers. The doses of the two tricyclics may be adjusted up or down, depending on John's headaches and side effects.

Sample Case History: Frequent Migraine Plus Severe Chronic Daily Headache and Menstrual Migraine

Sally is a 45-year-old woman with two migraines per week and severe daily headaches. She usually has 1 day of severe migraine the first day of her menses, but she has irregular menstrual periods. Sally has mild insomnia and a moderate anxiety disorder. She is chronically mildly depressed, with a family history of depression. Her stomach is very sensitive to aspirin or NSAIDs.

With frequent migraines and severe daily headaches, we definitely want to utilize preventive medication. As usual, all of the nonmedication strategies are discussed with Sally, such as diet, relaxation exercises, etc. Amitriptyline (Elavil) is a logical first choice of preventive medication, because of Sally's insomnia, anxiety, migraines, and daily headaches. Amitriptyline is inexpensive and may help all of these conditions. It may decrease her mild depression, but we plan on using it in very low doses that are not as large as the usual antidepressant doses. We start with 10 mg at night, increasing to 25 mg each night after 4 nights. I give samples of 10 mg and 25 mg amitriptyline, and if patients have trouble with the 10 mg, I instruct them to simply stay on that low dose. I write in the chart that other preventive possibilities include: increasing amitriptyline, using nortriptyline if fatigue is too much of a problem, adding verapamil or a beta blocker (watching out for increased depression), fluoxetine (Prozac), or even phenelzine (Nardil). Clonazepam (Klonopin) at night sometimes will help both the insomnia and headaches, but is habit forming.

Thus, we begin the prevention program with amitriptyline. As an abortive, I give Sally Midrin or Fioricet (Esgic) for the migraines, because these are mild on the GI tract and she easily experiences GI upset. I also give her 20 mg of prednisone to take only for severe menstrual migraines, up to four tablets per month at most; these are dosed at one pill twice a day, as needed. She is to take this with food and Tums (or another antacid). I instructed her not to chase after the daily headaches with pain medicine, but that one or two Aspirin Free Excedrin (acetaminophen plus caffeine) is OK, two a day at most. I mark in the chart that other abortive possibilities include Anaprox, but she may have GI troubles with this, or DHE as an injection or nasal spray. Sumatriptan is a possibility.

Sally calls 2 weeks later, with improvement in daily headaches but continuing with two migraines per week. Her sleeping is improved, but she has a slightly dry mouth. I increase the dose of amitriptyline to 50 mg at night. The Midrin does not help, but Fioricet is helpful for her migraines.

One month later, Sally is in the office with a pulse of 100. The menstrual headaches do respond to prednisone, but she is nauseated with this medication. The daily headaches are significantly improved, but the migraines are not. At this point, I add a small amount of atenolol (Tenormin), 25 mg each night for 4 nights, then going up to one of the 50 mg tablets. This should decrease the migraines and offset the tachycardia of amitriptyline. I warn her about depression with atenolol, as she is chronically depressed. She is less depressed since being on 50 mg of amitriptyline. Sally states that Aspirin Free Excedrin helps, but she uses five a day. This is a danger sign that she may be climbing into the rebound situation with the caffeine, and I tell her to simply take nothing for the daily headaches. If patients understand the rebound situation, they usually will comply with this. However, many patients injest large amounts of OTC medications and never admit it to the physician. During this visit I draw a routine blood test, c.b.c. and SMA, because of the daily medication. I add 10 mg of metoclopramide (Reglan) to take with prednisone for nausea. She is instructed to take the prednisone with food and Tums.

Six weeks later, the atenolol and amitriptyline combination has diminished the migraines by 75%, but Sally is gaining weight. It can be very difficult to determine whether it is the antidepressant causing weight gain or the beta blocker. The amitriptyline is decreased to 25 mg at night, but the weight gain continues. We now stop the amitriptyline, and the headaches increase but the weight gain ceases. Unfortunately, we very often need to make compromises between side effects and efficacy of medication. Some patients cannot function with their daily headaches, and will tolerate annoying side effects such as constipation, dry mouth, fatigue, or weight gain. With most patients we attempt to search for a preventive medication that will minimize side effects. Compromising between the headaches and overuse of medication is a common process.

At this point, Sally is only on atenolol, with her daily headaches returning while off of the amitriptyline, but the migraines are significantly improved. We now add fluoxetine (Prozac), one-half capsule worth (in juice) each morning for 4 days, then one capsule each morning. Sally calls in 3 weeks, and her daily headaches are somewhat improved and her chronic low-level depression is much better. On the beta blocker (Atenolol) and fluoxetine, her anxiety is also improved. She does not sleep as well, and is up intermittently throughout the night. The decision at this point is whether to add more medication, such as a small amount of clonazepam (Klonopin) at night, or whether to leave the medication alone. Sally is not overly fatigued during the day, and thus we leave the insomnia alone, and do not add medication. The decision whether to add more medicine is a joint one between the physician and patient. If Sally stated that everything (the daily headaches and migraines, as well as the depression) was much better, but that she could not tolerate the insomnia, we might add a small amount of clonazepam. The amitriptyline was causing weight gain, so we effectively substituted fluoxetine (Prozac) for amitriptyline. Protriptyline (Vivactil) would be an alternative to fluoxetine, as protriptyline never causes weight gain.

Thus, at this point with Sally she is on atenolol at night, fluxetine in the morning, and she uses Fioricet (Esgic) or prednisone as abortives. Metoclopramide is taken with the prednisone for nausea. As always, the situation is subject to change with her medicines, and we may need to try DHE at some point, or we may want to increase atenolol or fluoxetine. Sumatriptan pills or injections are a good possibility. Keeping notes in the chart of other possibilities that apply to Sally renders future medication changes much easier.

Sample Case History: Two Migraines per Month

James is a 32-year-old male with a history of, on average, two very severe migraines per month, and one mild or moderate migraine per month. He does not experience an aura. As with most patients, the headaches may increase or decrease in certain months or seasons, and James has more severe headaches in spring and in the very humid days of summer. He only occasionally has nausea that bothers him. On my initial headache questionnaire, I always ask if the nausea bothers the patient, because some patients do not want the nausea treated. They feel better after vomiting, and state that the pain is the overwhelming problem. Others state that the nausea bothers them very much, and that they wish to have antiemetics available. The length of James's typical severe migraine varies from 5 to 24 hours, but averages closer to 5 hours. He needs to be able to work during his migraines, and cannot afford to take a day off for the headaches. In general, there is a tremendous amount of lost work and school time due to migraines.

With two severe and one or two milder migraines per month, I usually would not resort to daily preventive medication. It is more appropriate to simply utilize abortive treatment. I discuss with James the possibility of giving himself an injection, either DHE or sumatriptan, but he is reluctant to do this. Most patients who have not been extensively treated for migraines would much rather try pills or suppositories than self-injections. I keep in mind that the injections, or a nasal spray of DHE, are a possibility for the future. Sumatriptan pills are always a possibility.

I give James Anaprox D.S. to take at the onset and repeat in 1 hour, if necessary. He may take as many as three per day, with food or Tums. He is warned about GI side effects. I tell James that combining Anaprox with caffeine may add to the effectiveness. Caffeine is utilized in the form of coffee, a soft drink, or one-half or one 100 mg No-Doz (or similar) caffeine tablet. If he can afford to go to sleep, which stops most migraines, we skip the caffeine. The advantages of the anti-inflammatories, such as Anaprox, is that they are nonsedating and nonaddicting. Most patients are able to function very well on anti-inflammatories.

In addition to Anaprox, I give James Midrin, to take one or two capsules at the onset (try 1 first), and then he may repeat one every 45 minutes or so, up to five per day. Midrin may be combined with Anaprox. I warn him about being very "spacy" or tired with Midrin. Some patients find that combinations of these first line abortives work very well, and Anaprox and Midrin may be combined. Midrin may also be combined with a butalbital compound, but fatigue may be a problem. The addition of caffeine to Midrin is often helpful.

James does well with Anaprox, but is fatigued with Midrin, and it does not help. However, he is nauseated with Anaprox. I add Reglan, 5 or 10 mg, to take with Anaprox, Tums, and food, or he may take Reglan 10 minutes prior to the Anaprox. Alternatively, we could use Compazine, 10 mg tablets or the long acting 10 or 15 mg spansules.

The Anaprox and Reglan help but are not completely effective. James states that they help the milder migraines very much, but the severe migraines are only 50% improved, and he still cannot work during the headache. He does not wish to try DHE or sumatriptan injections, and therefore we have several options: standard ergots (such as Cafergot), Norgesic Forte, butalbital compounds (such as Fiorinal), or narcotics. Alternative anti-inflammatories may help more than naproxen (Anaprox), but usually if naproxen does not help, other anti-inflammatories will not be effective. Fiorinal, Fioricet, Esgic, and Phrenilin have relatively few side effects, but these are habit forming. For James's headaches, he would not be taking these every day, and the addiction risk is minimal. However, the ergots are more likely to simply stop the headache, and he is young enough where we would like to try this approach.

I give James Cafergot pills to try, one or two at the onset, and then one every hour as needed; I tell him that if four are not stopping the headache, to take no more Cafergot for that day. He is to use ergots for only 1 day in a 4 day period. I have James take 10 mg of Reglan prior to the Cafergot. He becomes extremely nauseated and nervous with Cafergot. I have a compounding pharmacist compound the Cafergot PB suppositories, and instruct James to take one third of a suppository every 1 to 3 hours, as needed. Since we have been having difficulty obtaining certain products, such as Cafergot PB, compounding pharmacists have been invaluable for many patients. The Cafergot PB suppository helps his severe headaches, with minimal nausea, and he reports that he does need one half of a suppository. I begin with a small amount of Cafergot suppositories, usually one-third, and have the patients titrate the dose. The next step would have been a butalbital compound, such as Fiorinal. DHE nasal spray, to be formulated by the compounding pharmacist, would be another possibility. Although the nasal spray is not as effective as the DHE injections, many patients are reluctant to give themselves an injection. At some point, we may wish to utilize sumatriptan pills or injections with James.

Sample Case: Severe Refractive Migraines Plus Chronic Daily Headache

Joanne is a 43-year-old woman with a long history of severe CDH plus frequent very severe migraines, two per week on average, with only mild nausea. She also has irritable bowel syndrome. She does not have a sleep disorder.

Joanne has seen a variety of people for her headaches, including six neurologists, four internists, two ENT doctors, an allergist, four dentists, three chiropractors, and a napropath. Multiple nonmedication strategies have been unsuccessful, including physical therapy, diet therapy, and acupuncture. She has had biofeedback, which helps to a small degree, and has seen several psychotherapists, who have helped Joanne cope with the headaches. However, she is very frustrated and continues experiencing the severe headaches.

Joanne's situation is seen frequently. Whatever psychopathology may or may not be present, we are left with the need to treat these headaches. Although biofeedback, relaxation therapy, and psychotherapy may help in many situations, in fact they are usually unsuccessful treatments, and in the end we are left with medication as the only effective therapy.

Joanne has been refractive to the following preventive medications: tricyclic antidepressants (amitriptyline and many others), beta blockers, calcium blockers, anti-inflammatories, methysergide (Sansert), and combinations of the above. Prozac and Zoloft did not help. The primary considerations would be valproic acid (Depakote), MAO inhibitors (Phenelzine), IV DHE therapy, and amphetamines (Ritalin, Dexedrine).

With abortive medication, Joanne has tried virtually all sorts of migraine medications, many sedatives, and narcotics. She has not had DHE intramuscularly, nor has she had sumatriptan. Joanne has never tried corticosteroids, which I use in severe headache patients on a very limited basis.

Because of the above history, a stronger preventive approach is necessary. It is possible that no medication regimen will help Joanne, as a small percentage of severe headache patients are refractive to all medication possibilities. I give her four injections of IV DHE in the office (see section on IV DHE in Chapters 2 and 3) and begin phenelzine (Nardil), an MAOI. Valproate (Depakote) would possibly be a good choice, but phenelzine is more likely to help the CDH. If the headaches do not improve with the phenelzine alone, I may need to add a tricyclic antidepressant, such as nortriptyline, or a calcium blocker such as verapamil. However, adding medication increases possible side effects. I begin with one phenelzine (15 mg) each night, increasing to two after 4 days. Using the MAOI at night minimizes the risk of any food interactions. Joanne is counseled on the MAO diet and told to avoid Demerol, OTC cold medications, and to call my office before going on any new medication. I give her 10 mg capsules of Procardia to bite or cut and put under her tongue for any phenelzine reaction. (See section on MAO inhibitors, Chapter 3.)

As an abortive, Joanne wishes to try DHE IM, as it is significantly less expensive than sumatriptan. The sumatriptan has less associated nausea, but Joanne has relatively little nausea with her migraines. Sumatriptan is not to be used with MAOIs. She is asked to refrain from consuming pain medications or OTC medications.

Joanne responds well to the IV DHE (4 doses), and the severity of the daily headaches decreases by 50%. The migraines are also more manageable. IM DHE helps to a moderate degree, although she is not happy about giving herself an injection, and saves them for use as a last resort. I give her Thorazine suppositories, 100 mg, to use for a severe migraine, in order to sedate her and to avoid an emergency room visit. I also give Joanne prednisone, 20 mg tablets, to take as needed, twice a day, up to three tablets per month only. Decadron could also be utilized, and may be more effective than prednisone.

Two weeks later, I see Joanne; she is on the two Nardil per night, with no side effects, but the headaches are not improved. In the office, she is not orthostatic. Prednisone helped the severe migraines, and Thorazine did allow her to go to sleep, but she was "knocked out" the next day. I ask her to cut the Thorazine suppository in half, for a total of 50 mg of Thorazine. The IM DHE, prednisone, and Thorazine have kept Joanne from going to the emergency room. The severe anticipation of a migraine is frightening to many patients, and knowing medications are available that can help when they do get the headache is very reassuring to them.

At this point, I increase the phenelzine (Nardil) to three 15 mg tablets at night. Adding verapamil (Calan, Isoptin) or nortriptyline (Pamelor, Aventyl) are possibilities. The risks and problems of adding tricyclics to MAOIs are discussed in the section on MAOIs in Chapter 3.

Ten days later, I speak to Joanne on the phone. The headaches are the same, and she has no side effects from the phenelzine. At this point, I add one more phenelzine in the morning, for a total of four in the day. Two weeks later, she states that the headaches are much improved, but she is not sleeping. Insomnia and weight gain are common side effects with the MAOIs, and these side effects often lead to discontinuation of the medicine. However, in Joanne's case, she has been refractive to multiple medications, and we decide to treat the insomnia. I switch the phenelzine to two in the morning and two in the afternoon. At night, I add Klonopin (generic = clonazepam), 0.5 mg each night. The alternate choices would be tricyclics that are sedating, such as amitriptyline, nortriptyline, or doxepin. However, Klonopin often helps the headaches, and is less of a problem in combination with phenelzine.

Joanne is now on four phenelzine during the day and 0.5 mg Klonopin at night. She does well, but 2 months later the headaches begin to break through. We could add verapamil or a tricyclic, but at this point I revert back to IV DHE, which helped in the beginning. I give Joanne four injections in the office, 1 mg each. This greatly decreases the headaches, but 3 weeks later both the migraines and daily headaches are increasing again. However, Joanne states that she has been able to work and function much better since being on Nardil. She feels that the Klonopin also helps her headaches. Her blood pressure is slightly lower than her baseline, but she is not orthostatic. At this point I would add nortriptyline (Pamelor), 10 mg each night. Fatigue, weight gain, insomnia, and dry mouth may all become problems. With phenelzine and a tricyclic antidepressant, the blood pressure may decrease to a point where the patient becomes symptomatic.

If patients have side effects on MAOIs, we can either treat the side effects with more drugs, or we can decrease the amount of medication. Usually, I decrease the amount of the MAOI or stop it altogether. However, very severe, refractive headache patients welcome the headache relief that they may receive. Occasionally, side effects may be treated with more medication, as is the case with insomnia. Weight gain is difficult to treat, and a diuretic may buy some more time on the MAOI, but usually the weight gain continues, and the phenelzine needs to be lowered or discontinued altogether. Orthostatic hypotension with these medications is best treated by lowering medication; an alternative is adding fludrocortisone acetate (Florinef), 0.1 mg once or twice a day. However, this usually leads to edema, and is unlikely to be tolerated in the long term. Although we do not like to treat side effects with more medication, these patients are desperate, and the relief that they receive from medications such as MAOIs may be the first break from headaches that they have sustained in years.

With Joanne, I add nortriptyline, 10 mg each night. After 2 weeks, the headaches are milder, and we continue on the medication regimen of four phenelzine tablets during the day and 10 mg of nortriptyline and 0.5 mg of Klonopin at night. We could stop the Klonopin and observe how her sleeping is without it. With headache medications, we always want to minimize medication but maximize effectiveness. In the future, with Joanne, I may increase the tricyclic (nortriptyline), change to valproic acid (Depakote), or add a small amount of verapamil (Isoptin, Calan). Amphetamines would also be a consideration as an "end of the line" therapy.

Sample Case: Analgesic Rebound Headache in a Patient with Severe, Frequent Migraines and Severe Daily Headaches

Mark is a 23-year-old man with a history, since age 5, of severe daily headaches and frequent migraines, once to twice per week. As with most patients with a history of severe headaches since early childhood, these are headaches that he inherited from both sides of his family. If both parents have had migraines, usually all of the children will have headaches. He has been refractive to the usual first line preventive medications, including tricyclic antidepressants, Prozac, verapamil, beta blockers, and NSAIDs. He takes 12 to 14 pills per day of an aspirin and caffeine combination. Mark has noticed that the headaches have increased in severity as his analgesic consumption has accelerated.

The usual migraine teachings need, of course, to be done with Mark: diet, not to miss meals, wear sunglasses outside, and to utilize ice packs where the headache hurts. I instruct Mark to watch his neck posture so that his cervical spine is in a neutral position; it is important to have students or office workers raise up the level of their desk so that the neck is not as flexed. Utilizing a speaker phone, instead of bending the neck on the telephone, helps some patients avoid neck pain. Neck stretching exercises may help.

Relaxation or biofeedback is offered to Mark, as is a program of "headache-stress management," incorporating stress management techniques with, if applicable, psychotherapy or cognitive therapy. Some patients welcome a more holistic approach, and others wish to only use medication. Combining the two approaches is ideal.

Mark is in the analgesic rebound situation, with an increase in headaches from the aspirin and caffeine combination. His true headache pattern, or severity of his underlying migraines and daily headaches, is unknown at this point because of the rebound situation. It is a fallacy to pretend, in this rebound situation, that the offending drug being overused is the only cause of the headaches, because there was a reason why the patient took that drug in the first place. Once we stop the drug responsible for the rebound, and we are over the rebound situation, the true headache severity will be seen. The severity of the underlying headaches is, in my experience, usually 25% to 75% less after the rebound headaches are stopped. However, a significant number of people do not appreciably decrease their headaches by stopping the analgesics, and the rebound headache situation does not actually apply to them.

The strategy with Mark is to withdraw the offending drug causing rebound, in this case an aspirin and caffeine preparation, and to institute effective preventive medication. We need to educate Mark as to the dangers of constantly "chasing" after the headaches all day. There are generally two manners in which the rebound drug may be withdrawn: all at once (cold turkey) or slowly. It is often necessary to simply throw away all of the offending medicine, for if it is in the house, the patient will take it. Mark's situation is not as difficult as the situation with an addicting sedative or narcotic, because the withdrawal is usually milder with aspirin and caffeine. Many patients taking butalbital or narcotic preparations originally take the medication for daily headaches, and then increase their use as they realize that the medication helps stress, depression, anxiety, and gives them an "energy boost" for several hours.

Mark decides that he must stop the medication abruptly, because if it is in his apartment, he will take the aspirin and caffeine. I estimate that he is consuming the equivalent of 12 cups of coffee per day through the medication, and I urge him to not abruptly stop all of the caffeine. The caffeine withdrawal headache can be very severe, and many patients suffer through this withdrawal on weekends, when they abruptly decrease their caffeine. He agrees to consume several cups of coffee or cans of soda per day, so as not to immediately shut off the caffeine. With medication, Mark has been refractive to all of the first line preventive medications. It may be worthwhile to utilize one of the first line medications again, because when patients are in the analgesic rebound situation, they may be refractive to all medications used to prevent headaches. Medications that patients seemed resistant to are often effective after the analgesics are discontinued.

We decide to use a second line preventive medication, valproate (Depakote). Later, if we need to, we could add a first line medication such as amitriptyline or propranolol. If we can keep Mark from overusing analgesics, the first line medications that were previously ineffective may indeed help. We begin with one Depakote, 250 mg, twice a day, with food. The plan will be to increase this dose to 1,000 or 2,000 mg per day, if necessary. Many patients improve on as little as 250 or 500 mg of Depakote. As with most preventives, at least 3 weeks needs to be allowed for the Depakote to work. A c.b.c. and an SMA need to be drawn at least once in the first month.

Along with using the Depakote, we stop the aspirin and caffeine. I ask Mark to continue some caffeine, the equivalent of three cups of coffee. If he simply stops all caffeine, a severe withdrawal migraine may ensue. I give Mark four injections of IV DHE, over 2 days, in the office. This can be accomplished in the office with much more convenience for the patient than the hospital. At the same time, we teach Mark how to use DHE as an IM injection.

Mark does well for the 2 days on DHE, but after this he begins to have severe daily headaches. We are now in the rebound situation; the Depakote has not had a chance to work, and his basic underlying headache pattern is also very severe. I give him four pills of prednisone, 20 mg each, to take one each day. The headaches are slightly improved over these 4 days. I speak with him frequently, and encourage him not to retreat back to the aspirin and caffeine. If patients understand the reason behind stopping pain medication, I find that they are much more likely to follow the program. I give him 10 mg prochlorperazine (Compazine) tablets or 25 mg suppositories to help with the nausea of the migraines, and to decrease the nausea from his DHE injections. He finds that DHE helps, but he is nauseated and has mild leg cramps from the injections. Antiemetic medication is very helpful in providing sedation, as well as in combating the nausea. Compazine is effective, but some patients become agitated or restless with this antiemetic. Promethazine (Phenergan), although more sedating and less effective, rarely creates anxiety.

Mark manages to stay off of the aspirin and caffeine, but he begins to call for pain medications. Some patients, in this rebound situation, need a sedative to weather the withdrawal; in other patients we simply do not want to begin with pain medication or addicting sedative medication. If sedatives, such as diazepam (Valium), are given, they need to be limited, and given for only 1 to 3 weeks. I increase Mark's Depakote to 500 mg twice a day, and ask him to refrain from using pain medication. At the 3 week point, he has had a rough time, but the headaches are definitely less than when he was on the aspirin and caffeine. He is having mild to moderate daily headaches, and one migraine in the past week that was decreased with IM DHE. Blood tests are normal; I usually do not test the level of valproate until we progress to 1,500 mg per day. Because of nausea, I substitute sumatriptan for the DHE. This works well for Mark.

The headaches remain tolerable, but after several months Mark has gained 8 pounds, is beginning to lose hair, and is very fatigued on the Depakote. All of these side effects are occasionally seen with Depakote. We decide to stop the Depakote, and see how he does with no preventive medication. As abortives, Mark has sumatriptan injections and Compazine, and we add Midrin as a milder abortive medication.

One week after stopping Depakote, he reports severe daily headaches again. At this point, we have several choices: (1) retry a first line medication, (2) methysergide (Sansert), and (3) phenelzine (Nardil). The first line medications have not been effective with Mark, and are unlikely to help now. We proceed with methysergide (2 mg), one each day with food. We warn Mark about the need for stopping this medication every 5 or 6 months. I also warn him that he may feel terribly ill from Sansert, with nausea, stomach upset, leg cramps, heat flashes about the head, sweats, etc. If patients are aware of the severe side effects, they do not panic when these occur with Sansert.

Mark notices that the migraines are decreased on one Sansert, but the daily headaches remain severe. We go up to two Sanserts, but the daily headaches do not decrease in severity. The idea with Sansert is always to keep the dose as low as possible. Occasionally, I will go up to four or five pills per day. In the hope of avoiding phenelzine (Nardil), I add protriptyline (Vivactil), a nonsedating tricyclic that is helpful for daily headaches. Vivactil almost never causes weight gain, and fatigue is rare. The anticholinergic side effects, such as dry mouth, constipation, and blurred vision, may be severe. We start with one 5 mg pill of Vivactil each morning. Many patients cannot tolerate more than one-half or one 5 mg tablet per day of protriptyline.

Mark reports that the headaches are not improved, and we push the Vivactil to 10 mg, one tablet twice a day. The daily headaches are slightly better. At this point, the decision is whether to stop the Vivactil and progress to an MAOI (Nardil). In younger patients such as Mark, I always attempt to avoid the MAOIs, but they can be very effective. Weight gain and insomnia often become major problems, however. Mark is improved on this regimen of Sansert and Vivactil, and we decide to compromise. Often, we need to strike a balance between headaches and medication. In striving to improve headaches, we risk overmedicating. How much medication to use depends upon the severity of headaches and the patient's willingness to risk side effects of medicine. The patient plays a crucial role in this decision. If we progress to Nardil plus a tricyclic or Nardil plus verapamil, the patient first needs to know the problems associated with this regimen.

With Mark, we decide to hold the line on further medication, and continue to use the Vivactil, Sansert, and sumatriptan. Midrin has not helped, and we stop this medication. The next step would be to increase Sansert and/or Vivactil, or to stop Vivactil and begin an MAOI (Nardil). Nardil and Sansert may be used together. Sumatriptan cannot be used with Nardil. In the future, with Mark, we may be using the MAOI, but at the moment we decide to stay with the Sansert and Vivactil. If Mark begins to use pain medications again, he will undoubtedly slip back into the rebound headache situation.

CHAPTER 6

Introduction to Tension Headache and Tension Headache Abortive Medication

Tension headache is perhaps not the best choice of terms for this type of headache because it implies that tension in people's lives is the cause of the headache. Although stress and tension in one's life tend to increase headache, they are not usually the cause of the headaches, but simply an exacerbating factor. When the headaches occur daily, a better term is chronic daily headache (CDH).

Clinical Features of Tension Headache

The pain of tension headache may occur anywhere about the cranium, but it is usually bilateral, and described as bandlike, aching, pressing, tightening, or dull. The severity is usually mild or moderate, and often waxes and wanes throughout the day. Some patients do experience severe daily headaches. As many as 10% to 15% of tension headache patients awaken from 1 to 6 a.m. with a headache that is often pounding or throbbing in nature. Neck pain may accompany tension headache, but is seen no more often than with migraine headache.

Tension headache may begin at any age, but in 40% of patients it begins in childhood or adolescence. When both parents have had migraine or daily headache, and the child has had daily headaches for several years, the headaches will often continue for a lifetime. Tension headache may remit for months or years, or disappear completely. The course is very difficult to predict in any one person.

The majority of patients with tension headache also experience periodic migraine headaches, which vary in frequency from patient to patient. In some patients, the tension headache is much more of a problem than is the migraine, and the tension headaches are treated accordingly. Alternatively, patients may state that they do not mind the daily headaches, but that the severe migraines are what truly bother them the most, and we adjust the medication to attack the migraines, not the tension headaches.

Dizziness, nausea, and sensitivity to bright lights may accompany the tension headache in some patients, and at times it is very difficult to distinguish the more severe tension headache from a milder migraine. We are possibly viewing a spectrum of one illness, with tension headache at the milder end and migraine being more severe. Many patients with a history of migraine develop daily headaches. (See Table 6.1).

Although tension headache is usually not severe, vast numbers of people suffer with a daily, aggravating or annoying headache (CDH); they awaken with it and they go to sleep with it. The overuse of analgesics to fight these daily headaches is costly, both in terms of side effects and money. Many patients increase their headaches by overusing analgesics, because this leads to rebound headaches the next day. It is not unusual to encounter patients who take five to 20 pills of an OTC preparation on a daily basis, and this may go on for years or decades. Analgesic overuse may lead to stomach, liver, or renal problems. The strategy with patients who require daily painkillers in excess is to decrease the analgesics and to institute relaxation methods and/or preventive medication.

Sinus and TMJ Disorders

Sinus pathology can complicate the picture with migraine and tension headache. Frontal "dull" head pain may, at times, be lessened by decongestants and/or cortisone-based nasal sprays. Patients with chronically congested sinuses often undergo surgery on the sinuses; at times, this may lessen headache. Further complicating the issue is the fact that cold or sinus medication may help any type of headache in certain patients.

It is important to inquire about bruxism, as a bite splint may be very helpful in some patients. The palpation of facial muscles may reveal hypertrophy and/or tenderness. Exquisite tenderness in the involved muscles, particularly the lateral pterygoids, suggests that a referral to a TMJ specialist may be in order. An abnormal exam of the temporomandibular joint, in conjunction with symptoms relating to the joint (such as locking), should also prompt a referral.

Pathophysiology of Tension Headache

The pathophysiology of tension headache remains uncertain; however, it is likely that increased muscular tension, vascular changes, and primary CNS differences all play a role. Research has indicated that many of the differences found in the bloodstream and CNS of migraine patients are also found in those with tension headaches. It is difficult to locate sufficient daily tension headache patients who do not have migraine in order to do adequate studies. In both tension and migraine patients it is possible to locate areas of scalp or cervical tenderness by palpation, but this muscle tension and tenderness is most likely the result of processes beginning in the CNS.

TABLE 6.1. Links Connecting Tension and Migraine Headache.

Both respond to similar medications: antidepressants, verapamil, anti-inflammatories, and beta blockers.
Similar serotonergic changes are found in tension and migraine headache patients.
Neck pain and muscle spasm are common to both tension and migraine.
Family history of headache is present in both migraine and tension headache patients.
Prevalence of epilepsy is increased in tension and migraine.
Cranial muscle tenderness and cerebral blood flow changes are common to both conditions.
Mild migraine is very difficult to clinically distinguish from a severe tension headache.
The vast majority of patients with CDH also experience migraine.

Psychological factors may contribute to the presence of tension headache, but there is no consistent evidence that tension headache patients truly have more psychiatric disorders than patients without headache. Various studies have revealed high rates of depression, anxiety, or a history of abuse as children in patients with CDH, but other studies have revealed conflicting results. Although headache is a feature of depression in some patients, depression as a cause of headache has generally been overstated. Patients often become depressed about having daily headaches or severe migraines, and when the headaches are adequately treated, the depression may lessen. Unresolved anger and psychological stresses undoubtedly do contribute to headache. However, it is generally a mistake to overemphasize psychological factors with patients. Most headache patients are very frustrated by attempts to resolve their headache through nonmedicine avenues. See Chapter 1 for a discussion of psychological factors and relaxation methods in headache.

Treatment of Tension Headache

The two most consistently helpful methods for decreasing tension headache are medication and relaxation methods. Psychotherapy and stress management are helpful in some patients. At times, physical therapy, massage, or chiropractic therapy are useful, particularly with severe increased cervical muscle tension. Ice is usually useful for any type of headache, and some patients find that heat also helps. Acupuncture has not been proven to be more effective than placebo. With the overwhelming majority of tension headache patients, medication is easily the most effective treatment, and relaxation/biofeedback is also helpful for some of these patients. Most patients are unwilling to learn and practice relaxation, and if they do learn it, the number of patients who continue to do the relaxation over time is small.

Relaxation Therapy for Tension Headache

Relaxation may be learned at home, with minimal cost. Most patients may learn the simple deep breathing techniques and imaging by utilizing cassette tapes and booklets on relaxation. Patients need to be encouraged to do the deep breathing intermittently throughout the day, particularly when a stressful time arises. As little as 20 seconds of deep breathing, done slowly, may be enough to prevent the headache from increasing. I encourage patients to try to do the relaxation, even for just 20 seconds, instead of automatically reaching for a pill. If patients are encouraged to refrain from constantly taking pain medication and to simply utilize the relaxation, we often are able to decrease analgesic consumption. The rebound headache situation with analgesic overuse is a major cause of increased severity and frequency of headaches.

Some patients, particularly children, cannot learn relaxation by themselves at home, or they become frustrated with it. We then utilize formal relaxation or biofeedback training, at times with the biofeedback instrumentation. However, the cost of biofeedback programs has prevented many patients from attempting the relaxation/biofeedback, and simple home-based programs allow many more patients to utilize these nonmedication methods. In general, the younger the patient, the more successful the relaxation program will be. Motivation plays a key role in the success of relaxation. I strongly encourage children (after age 8) and adolescents to try the relaxation methods. See Chapter 1 and Appendix E for a discussion of relaxation techniques.

Medication for Tension Headache

As with other types of headache, we utilize abortive and preventive medications for tension headache. For most patients with episodic tension headaches, abortive medications are all that are required. However, if patients need to take analgesics very frequently, and are bothered more than minimally by CDH, preventive medicine should be instituted. The decision as to whether to use daily preventive medicines depends upon many factors, including the following: (1) severity of the tension headaches, (2) frequency and severity of coexisting migraines, and (3) the amount of analgesics being consumed. Many patients do not wish to be on daily medication, and they tend to ignore their mild daily headaches. Others are terribly bothered by the daily tension headaches and feel that they greatly decrease their quality of life. In these patients, an aggressive approach with daily prophylactic medication is indicated. Most patients do wish to utilize abortive medication, even when they are on preventive medications.

Abortive Medication

Our goal with tension headache abortive medication is to decrease the pain with the mildest possible medication. I try and minimize abortive medications, and I encourage patients to try taking six deep breaths, for 20 or 30 seconds, prior to reaching for the analgesics, or to simply attempt to ignore mild daily pain. We do not want patients to "chase" after the pain all day with analgesics, and if they need to do this, preventive medication should be utilized. With the overuse of analgesics, the rebound headache situation often becomes a problem.

In general, we avoid addicting medications for tension headache, except if the first line (nonaddicting) medications are ineffective. The only situation where daily addicting medications are justified for headache is when other avenues have failed. In elderly patients, some of the narcotic medications have less side effects than the preventives and nonaddicting analgesics; therefore, in this age group, addicting painkillers are, at times, utilized on a daily basis.

The first line abortive medications begin with the OTC analgesics. Ibuprofen and aspirin tend to be more effective than acetaminophen. Caffeine adds to the analgesia, and sometimes the caffeine itself is all that is needed. Caffeine, either alone or in combination with aspirin or acetaminophen, needs to be limited, so as to avoid rebound headaches.

OTC first line medications for tension headache include the following: acetaminophen, aspirin, caffeine, caffeine plus aspirin or acetaminophen combinations (such as Excedrin E.S., Aspirin Free Excedrin, and Anacin), and ibuprofen. Prescription first line medications for tension headache include: naproxen (Naprosyn, Anaprox), flurbiprofen (Ansaid), Midrin, and Norgesic Forte.

If the above first line medications are not effective, and preventive medication is not utilized, the addicting analgesics and benzodiazepines may be used. These need to be limited and monitored, and should only be used for moderate to severe pain. The addicting medications comprise the second line abortive medications for tension headache; they include: butalbital compounds (Fiorinal, Fioricet, Esgic, Phrenilin), narcotics, and benzodiazepines.

First Line Abortive Medication

Acetaminophen

Although acetaminophen is not very effective for most people with severe headaches, it is useful for milder headache. Aspirin or ibuprofen are usually more effective. Side effects to acetaminophen are minimal, and it may be used during pregnancy, as well as in patients with gastritis or ulcer disease.

The usual dose for acetaminophen is one or two "extra strength" tablets, 500 or 650 mg each, every 3 or 4 hours, limited to six of the pills per day. Do not exceed 4 g per day. Ingestions of 5 to 8 g per day, over weeks, have resulted in liver damage. Some patients consume 5 to 10 g of

TABLE 6.2. Quick Reference Guide: First Line Tension Abortive Medications.

1. Acetaminophen, Aspirin: These are the staples of OTC pain relief; acetaminophen is much less effective for headache, but better tolerated. These need to be limited, so as to avoid the rebound situation.
2. Ibuprofen (Motrin): Helpful for migraine and tension headache. Useful in children, and a liquid form is available. GI upset is relatively common, but ibuprofen is more effective for headache than acetaminophen.
3. Caffeine: Caffeine beverages or tablets (100 mg) are helpful for migraine and tension headache, either alone or as an adjunct to analgesics. Caffeine added to other abortives enhances their effectiveness and decreases drowsiness. For example, Midrin plus caffeine is an effective combination.
4. Caffeine-aspirin combinations: Excedrin (E.S.) has 65 mg of caffeine, 250 mg of aspirin, and 250 mg of acetaminophen; this is a very effective OTC preparation, but overuse leads to rebound headaches. Anacin contains much less caffeine (32 mg). Aspirin Free Excedrin is a very useful combination of acetaminophen and caffeine.
5. Naproxen (Anaprox D.S.): Useful in younger patients, nonsedating, but very frequent GI upset. The usual dose is one 550 mg Anaprox D.S. tablet with food, that may be repeated, up to a maximum of three per day. If used on a daily basis, two per day should be the limit.
6. Flurbiprofen (Ansaid): Ansaid is a well-tolerated anti-inflammatory, similar to ibuprofen or naproxen. Useful in migraine and menstrual migraine, as well as tension headache. The addition of caffeine to any anti-inflammatory enhances the effect. GI upset is common, but Ansaid is nonaddicting and not sedating. One tablet every 3 to 4 hours is the usual dose, with a limit of three, and occasionally four, per day.
7. Midrin: Effective, safe, and used in children as well as adults. Primarily a migraine abortive, Midrin is also very helpful for tension headache. The usual dose is one or two per day to start, then one every hour as needed, five or six per day at most. May be combined with caffeine for increased efficacy.
8. Norgesic Forte: Effective nonaddicting combination of aspirin, caffeine, and orphenadrine. GI side effects are common, as is fatigue. Usual dose is one-half or one tablet every 3 or 4 hours, four per day at most.

acetaminophen per day for years for their headaches. There is no limit to the numbers of OTC medications that desperate headache patients will swallow. Tubular necrosis, or even myocardial damage, may be a problem with chronic high dose acetaminophen.

Acetaminophen is available in suppositories, tablets (regular and chewable), wafers, capsules, an elixir, liquid, a solution, and as effervescent granules with sodium bicarbonate (Bromo Seltzer).

Aspirin

Aspirin has been the mainstay of headache therapy for many years, and remains an extremely helpful abortive. It is more effective for headaches than is acetaminophen, but carries an increased risk of side effects. Aspirin should be avoided during pregnancy or with gastritis or ulcer disease. The many side effects of aspirin are well known, and include bleeding from the GI tract, prolongation of the bleeding time, bruising, reversible hepatic damage, and exacerbation of rhinitis and bronchospasm. The usual dose is 325 to 650 mg every 4 hours, as needed.

Aspirin is available in many forms, including buffered tablets. The addition of a small amount of an antacid possibly increases the absorption and decreases the GI irritation.

Caffeine

Caffeine helps headaches via vascular effects, and possibly by increasing serotonin levels. Caffeine is very helpful for tension and migraine headaches. In addition, caffeine plays an important role in treating lumbar puncture headache. Overuse of caffeine may increase headaches via rebound mechanisms. Some patients do not suffer rebound headaches from 500 mg per day of caffeine, and others have rebound with as little as 30 mg. In general, I like to limit caffeine to 200 mg or, at most, 300 mg per day.

The average 8 ounce cup of coffee has 75 to 125 mg of caffeine. Drip coffee is stronger than percolated, and instant is the weakest form. Depending on size and strength, instant coffee may possess from 40 to 150 mg of caffeine, but is usually closer to 40 mg. Decaffeinated coffee has 2 to 5 mg per cup. These all depend upon the strength of the product and brew method.

Tea usually contains 30 to 50 mg per cup, and soft drinks average approximately 40 mg. Chocolate contains 1 to 15 mg per ounce, but cocoa has considerably more, up to 50 mg for 8 ounces.

Caffeine is available in food products and as tablets or capsules. Caffeine tablets, such as No Doz, Tirend, and Vivarin, are available in

TABLE 6.3. Caffeine: Sources and Strengths.

Limit to 200 mg per day, or, at most, 300 mg per day.
Coffee, 8 ounces
    Average cup: 75–125 mg of caffeine.
    Drip stronger than percolated, which is stronger than instant.
    Instant = 40–150 mg per cup, usually closer to 40 mg.
    Decaf = 2–5 mg per cup.
Tea (one cup)
    30–50 mg of caffeine per cup.
Soft drinks
    Approximately 40 mg per cup.
Chocolate
    1–15 mg per ounce.
Cocoa
    50 mg per 8 ounces.
Caffeine tablets that contain 100 mg of caffeine include: NoDoz, Vivarin, and Tirend.
Caffeine is present in many analgesic medications, such as Excedrin E.S., Anacin, and
    Vanquish.

100 mg forms. Higher strengths are available, but I do not use these. (See Table 6.3)

When patients find that caffeine significantly decreases their headache, I will occasionally utilize the pure caffeine tablets, with a dose of one half of a 100 mg pill every 3 to 4 hours, as needed. At times, it is helpful to combine caffeine with medications that do not contain caffeine, such as Midrin.

Whatever manner that patients receive caffeine, whether in coffee, caffeine pills, or combination analgesics, we need to limit the total amount of caffeine. The maximum amount per day varies from person to person, depending upon their sleep patterns, presence of anxiety, and sensitivity to possible rebound headaches.

Combinations of Aspirin (or Acetaminophen) Plus Caffeine

We increase the efficacy of analgesics by adding caffeine; the primary problem with these medications is the risk of rebound headaches. However, when used in moderation, the combination analgesics are very helpful in treating both tension and migraine headaches.

There are many medications that contain combinations of aspirin and caffeine, or aspirin plus acetaminophen plus caffeine. I have chosen Excedrin E.S., Aspirin Free Excedrin, and Anacin as examples. However, there are numerous others that are comparable, such as: Saleto, Presalin, Trigesic, Salatin, S-A-C Tablets, Supac, Tri-Pain, Buffets II, Duradyne, Vanquish, BC Tablets, Anodynos, Cope, Midol, and BC Powder. For some patients, the powdered aspirin and caffeine combinations are more effective than the tablets.

Extra-Strength Excedrin

Although it is a very effective OTC preparation of acetaminophen (250 mg), aspirin (250 mg), and caffeine (65 mg), Excedrin E.S. should be used cautiously on a daily basis, as it can cause rebound headaches, as well as increase the risk for renal complications. The increased caffeine renders Excedrin more effective than most of the OTC preparations.

If Excedrin is used on a daily basis, the limit should be two per day, with occasional exceptions. If patients require more than this amount, consideration should be given to daily prevention medication.

The usual dose is one or two tablets every 3 or 4 hours, as needed, and the total dose per day, week, and month needs to be limited. Nausea or anxiety are common with aspirin and caffeine. Long term use may predispose to renal problems, or gastric irritation and bleeding.

Aspirin Free Excedrin

A useful combination of acetaminophen and caffeine, Aspirin Free Excedrin eliminates the GI side effects of aspirin. Although not as effective as Excedrin E.S., for patients with ulcers or GI upset this is a helpful product.

The usual dosage is two pills every 3 to 4 hours. This well tolerated medication seldom produces side effects other than the anxiety or insomnia from caffeine.

Anacin

Anacin caplets and tablets contain less caffeine than Excedrin E.S., and no acetaminophen. Anacin has 400 mg of aspirin and 32 mg of caffeine. Anacin Maximum Strength contains 500 mg of aspirin and 32 mg of caffeine. By decreasing the amount of caffeine, the efficacy declines, but we also limit side effects. With less caffeine, the rebound headache situation is less apt to be a problem. By eliminating acetaminophen, we decrease possible renal and hepatic toxicity. The usual dose of Anacin is one or two every 3 to 4 hours, as needed.

Ibuprofen (Motrin)

This OTC anti-inflammatory is beneficial for tension and migraine headaches. It is reasonably well tolerated. The relatively low cost and easy accessibility render ibuprofen very useful for tension headaches. Side effects, such as frequent GI upset, are similar to the other anti-inflammatories, such as naproxen. The dose varies from 200 mg (one pill of the OTC preparation) to 800 mg every 3 to 4 hours, as needed. The addition of caffeine may enhance efficacy. The total dose should not exceed 2,400 mg per day, and if ibuprofen is used daily, blood tests should be monitored with regularity. (See Chapter 2.)

Naproxen Sodium (Anaprox)

Each tablet of Anaprox DS contains 550 mg of naproxen sodium, a very effective anti-inflammatory for various types of headache. It is particularly useful around the menstrual period, and may be used as a preventive for migraine. Adding caffeine may increase the efficacy.

Nausea and GI upset are common. GI bleeding, liver toxicity, or renal damage may occur, and if naproxen is used on a daily basis, blood tests should be monitored.

Anaprox D.S. may be used up to three per day at 3 hour intervals. For migraine, the dosing is somewhat different, because we usually wish to use more naproxen in the first 1 to 2 hours. For tension headache, one tablet should be sufficient in a 3 hour period. Occasionally, patients do well with the smaller dose, Anaprox 275 mg. (See Chapters 2 and 3.)

Flurbiprofen (Ansaid)

Flurbiprofen is one of a slew of newer anti-inflammatories that is helpful for both migraine and tension headache. Flurbiprofen is reasonably well tolerated, with all of the usual side effects and precautions of the other anti-inflammatories. The usual dose is 100 mg every 3 to 4 hours as needed, with four per day being the most that one may use. When used on a daily basis, flurbiprofen may prevent headaches, but blood tests need to be monitored. The tablets are available in 50 and 100 mg sizes.

Midrin

An effective, well tolerated medication, Midrin consists of a vasocon-strictor, isometheptane, combined with dichloralphenazone, a nonaddict-ing sedative, and 250 mg of acetaminophen. Midrin is primarily a migraine abortive, but it is effective for many patients with tension headache. Midrin may be given to children and the elderly. Adding caffeine helps offset the fatigue that is often felt with Midrin, and may decrease the headache pain. (See Chapter 2.)

The usual dose is one or two capsules to start, and then one every hour as needed. Limits of five per day and 20 per week should be given. The capsules are large, and they may be taken apart for children's use. The generic Midrin is not as effective as the brand name; this is the situation with many pain medications for headache.

Fatigue or mild GI upset are common. Many patients complain of feeling lightheaded or "spacy." Midrin can raise the blood pressure, and must be used very cautiously in patients with hypertension. (See Chapter 2.)

Norgesic Forte

Another aspirin and caffeine combination, Norgesic Forte, also con-tains orphenadrine, a nonaddicting muscle relaxant. Orphenadrine is also an antihistamine. Norgesic Forte is one of the strongest nonaddicting abortive medications for tension or migraine headache. The tablets con-tain 50 mg of orphenadrine, 770 mg of aspirin, and 60 mg of caffeine.

The usual dose is one-half or one pill every 3 to 4 hours, as needed. Many patients can only tolerate one half of a pill at one time. I usually limit the Norgesic Forte to three pills per day at most.

Nausea or fatigue are common. Lightheadedness or "spaciness" are also seen. Blurred vision may occur because of the orphenadrine. The large amount of aspirin is very irritating to the stomach. (See Chapter 2.)

Second Line Abortive Medication

For some patients, the first line abortives are not effective, and we need to progress on to stronger therapy. The addicting medications that are generally used are the butalbital compounds, the narcotics, or the benzodiazepines. These are discussed in Chapter 2 in the section on abortive medications for migraine. For patients who require medication

---

TABLE 6.4. Quick Reference Guide: Second Line Tension Headache Abortive Medications.

1. Butalbital compounds: Effective but habit forming. Fiorinal, Esgic, Esgic Plus, Fioricet, Axotal, and Phrenilin are the primary butalbital compounds. Generic butalbital preparations do not work as well as brand names. Sedation or euphoria are common. Limit the total per month, and strict limits need to be set. If used daily, one or two is the usual limit.
2. Narcotics: Codeine, hydrocodone, and propoxyphene are commonly utilized. These are a last resort, and should be limited per month, and generally should not be used on a daily basis. These need to be discontinued if patients use them to alleviate stress, depression, fatigue, or anxiety.
3. Sedatives: Most are benzodiazepines: diazepam (Valium) and clonazepam (Klonopin). Chlordiazepoxide (Librium) is also useful. Sedation is common. Because they are habit forming, these need to be monitored with a monthly limit. They are a last resort, not a first choice.

---

once per week or less, these medications do not pose a problem. However, for those who require daily, or almost daily, abortives, the habit forming medications may be troublesome. In some patients, preventive medication is not well tolerated, or is ineffective. In these patients, if the first line abortives are not effective, and relaxation therapy does not work, we may be left with the second line medications as the only alternative. We must be certain that patients are not using these medications to decrease stress, to give them more energy for several hours, or to aid their depression. When the patients use the addicting medications for these purposes, they often cross the line into chemical dependency. In the occasional patient, however, where all other means have failed, it may be justified to use limited amounts of habit forming medications on a daily basis.

Butalbital Compounds

These have been discussed at length in Chapter 2 in the section on abortive medications for migraine. These include Fiorinal, Axotal, Esgic, Esgic Plus, Fioricet, and Phrenilin. The ingredients differ for each of these compounds. In general, the generic butalbital compounds are not as effective as the brand names.

Narcotics and Sedatives

Narcotics have been reviewed in Chapter 2, and sedatives are discussed in Chapter 7.

The narcotics, such as codeine, hydrocodone, propoxyphene, etc., should only be used as an absolute last resort in patients with tension headaches. The need to use these on a daily basis is unusual, because most often the milder abortives are effective, or the daily preventives work well enough. Only when patients have failed other approaches, and their quality of life is significantly improved by narcotics, should these be used daily. Patients should not be using these for stress, depression, fatigue, or anxiety. Narcotics need to be limited and monitored.

The sedatives are primarily in the benzodiazepine class, and include (among others) diazepam (Valium) and clonazepam (Klonopin). Although we try to avoid daily use of these, at times this is justified. The idea is to keep the dose as low as possible, and to switch medications when the dose becomes excessive.

CHAPTER 7

Tension Headache Preventive Medication

Introduction

Tension headache is, perhaps, an unfortunate choice of terms because it implies that tension in the patient's life is at the root of the headache. Although stress and tension are important contributing factors toward daily headaches, they do not, by themselves, cause daily headaches. There needs to be a predisposition toward headache. The vast majority of patients with daily headaches also experience episodic migraine headaches.

There are two types of tension headache: episodic tension headache and chronic tension headache (chronic daily headache). The "as needed" abortive medications are essentially the same for the two types. When chronic daily headache (CDH) is more than mild, the preventive medication approach becomes very important. It is possible that tension-type headaches have an underlying pathophysiology similar to migraine, and we are simply observing different parts of a spectrum. It is clear that people are predisposed to these headaches, and the headaches are not simply a "psychological" problem. Although stress does affect tension headaches, just as stress affects most illnesses, it is unfair to tension headache sufferers to attribute their headaches to stress or psychological problems. Psychological approaches for headache patients are discussed in Chapter 1. Stress management and/or relaxation techniques should be introduced to these patients.

When patients require more than minimal amounts of daily abortive medication, we need to consider a prevention approach for the headaches. By continually using drugs containing aspirin and caffeine, or similar compounds, many patients increase their headaches by creating a rebound headache situation. The amount of daily analgesics that creates a rebound headache situation varies from person to person; with some patients, only two pills of aspirin and caffeine per day lead to a more severe headache the next day.

TABLE 7.1. Criteria for the Use of Prevention Medication.

1. The frequency and severity of the tension headaches significantly decreases the patient's quality of life.
2. The patient is willing to take daily medication, endure possible side effects, and change the medication, if necessary.
3. Abortive medications have not provided sufficient relief in small to moderate amounts, or the patient overuses analgesics because of the pain.

If the headaches cannot be "ignored", and are moderate to severe, it is usually best to utilize daily preventive medication. The decision as to which daily medication to use depends upon many factors, such as the presence and frequency of coexisting migraine, whether the patient sleeps well, the presence of gastritis, etc. Patients need to be aware of the possibility that the first preventive medication chosen may not be effective, and that we often need to try several preventives before achieving the goal of improving the pain with a minimum of side effects. Realistic goals need to be set prior to initiating preventive medication; I usually tell the patient that we are attempting to improve the headache situation 50% to 90%, while attempting to minimize medicine. We wish to achieve a compromise between the headaches and medication and not overmedicate the person. Most of the medications for headache have not received specific FDA indications for this use. The following is only a guide to what I consider reasonable and rational therapy for headache; prior to prescribing medications for patients, they need to be informed of, and accept, the complete set of contraindications and side effects as listed in the PDR and package insert.

Episodic Tension Headache

Episodic tension headaches are recurrent episodes of tension headache lasting minutes to days, but less than 15 per month, or 180 days per year. Many patients will suffer spells of daily tension headache for weeks or months, and then very little headache for a period of time. It is a very difficult question as to whether to classify these patients as having episodic or chronic tension headaches. As with migraines, these headaches may run seasonally.

For patients with episodic tension headaches, the abortive medication approach is usually all that is necessary. However, if patients are overusing "as needed" medications, and a rebound headache situation is suspected, preventive therapy may be beneficial. For abortive treatment of episodic tension headaches, see Chapter 6.

Chronic Tension Headache

This type of headache is present for at least 15 days a month for at least 6 months; when it is present on a daily basis, we refer to it as CDH (Chronic

TABLE 7.2. Quick Reference Guide: First Line CDH Prevention Medication.

1. Amitriptyline (Elavil): Effective and inexpensive. Helpful for migraines and daily headache. Sedation, dizziness, dry mouth, weight gain, and constipation are common. Important to begin with only 10 mg, as many patients cannot tolerate more than 10 mg.

2. Fluoxetine (Prozac): Fewer side effects than amitriptyline, but not as effective. Nausea, anxiety, insomnia are common. Weight gain may occur but is infrequent. Helpful for migraine in some patients. Begin with only 10 mg, as some patients cannot tolerate more than 10 mg/day. Expensive. Sertraline (Zoloft) is very similar.

3. Protriptyline (Vivactil): Effective and nonsedating. Weight gain does not occur. Dry mouth, constipation, dizziness are common. Used in the morning, as insomnia is a frequent side effect. May be used in the morning with a sedating tricyclic at night.

4. Nortriptyline (Pamelor, Aventyl): Better tolerated than amitriptyline, but less effective. Side effects are similar to amitriptyline, but less severe. Useful in children, adolescents, and the elderly. Occasionally helpful in migraine.

5. Doxepin (Sinequan): Very similar to amitriptyline; more effective than nortriptyline, but with increased side effects. Begin with very low doses (10 mg each night), as many patients cannot tolerate more than this amount.

6. NSAIDs: Not as effective as antidepressants for daily headache, but without the cognitive side effects. GI side effects are common, however. Hepatic and renal blood tests need to be monitored. NSAIDs are used more frequently in younger patients. Ibuprofen is available over the counter. Naproxen (Naprosyn, Anaprox) is more effective than ibuprofen. Flurbiprofen (Ansaid), diclofenac sodium (Voltaren), and ketoprofen (Orudis) are also utilized. As always, attempt to use the minimum effective dose.

Daily Headache). When the tension headaches are daily or very frequent, it is difficult to "chase" after them with abortive medications all day. When we do this, we risk creating rebound headaches. Many patients consume large amounts of OTC medication on a daily basis, with increased headaches as a result.

For CDH that is more than mild, or that bothers the patient to the point of interfering with the quality of his or her life, the preventive medication approach is instituted. Biofeedback and stress management have a role to play in some of these patients, and should be offered as a treatment option. Relaxation/biofeedback approaches are discussed in Chapter One. However, most patients who have moderate or severe daily headaches will benefit from a preventive medication approach.

First Line Preventive Therapy for CDH

The antidepressants are the mainstay of therapy for daily headaches. (See Table 7.4) They are effective whether or not the patient is depressed, and the reason that they help headaches is usually independent of anti-depressant action. The choice of which antidepressant to use depends

TABLE 7.3. Information That Patients Need to Know Prior to Starting Prevention Medication.

1. The realistic goals of the medication are to decrease the tension headache severity by 70%, not to completely eliminate the headaches. It is always wonderful when the headaches are 90% to 100% improved, but the idea is to minimize medication. Most patients need to be willing to settle for moderate improvement.
2. Patients must be willing to change medication, if necessary. They need to know that what is effective for somebody else may not work for them. Trial and error may be needed to find the best preventive approach for that person.
3. The preventive medication may take weeks to become effective, the doses often need to be adjusted, and thus patience will be necessary with these medications. The physician needs to be available for phone consultations pertaining to the headaches and medicine.
4. Most preventive medications are utilized in medicine for another purpose. It is best if patients are informed, for instance, that Elavil is also used for depression, usually in much higher doses. Patients should be told why we are utilizing Elavil, and that it is not because they are depressed.
5. Side effects are possible with any medication, and the patient has to be prepared to endure mild side effects in order to achieve results. We cannot simply stop medication and switch to another because of very mild side effects. Most patients are willing to put up with mild, annoying side effects.

upon many factors, including the anxiety level of the patient, whether there is a sleep disturbance, the age of the patient, and other medical conditions. If the patient has a tendency towards constipation, that also will influence our choice.

There are many antidepressants from which to choose, and not all are effective for headaches. The tricyclic antidepressants have been the most widely used for headaches, and are very effective. A newer medication, fluoxetine (Prozac) is rapidly gaining acceptance as a first line daily headache preventive. The most commonly used medication for daily headaches is amitriptyline.

Amitriptyline (Elavil)

The guidelines for using amitriptyline, as discussed in Chapter 3, apply to the use of amitriptyline as a daily headache preventive. Amitriptyline is particularly helpful for the associated insomnia that often accompanies daily headaches, and is beneficial in preventing accompanying migraines. Amitriptyline is the most effective tricyclic for migraine headaches, but for CDH the alternative antidepressants are often as effective. Amitriptyline is very inexpensive.

Despite the use of low doses, amitriptyline tends to be poorly tolerated by many patients. Amitriptyline is available in: 10, 25, 50, 75, 100, and 150 mg tablets. For a complete discussion of amitriptyline, see Chapter 3.

Fluoxetine (Prozac)

Fluoxetine has been a controversial medication with certain advantages over the older antidepressants because of its favorable side effect profile. Fluoxetine is the first of the selective serotonin reuptake inhibitors, and undoubtedly many more will follow. Sertraline (Zoloft) is a new medication similar to fluoxetine, with somewhat fewer side effects. Sertraline is discussed in the following section. Fluoxetine usually does not cause the dry mouth, weight gain, sedation, or constipation that is often seen with amitriptyline. We are justified in using fluoxetine as a first line daily headache preventive medication, particularly in patients with chronic low level depression. Fluoxetine is somewhat helpful in preventing migraine as well as daily headaches. Fluoxetine may be combined with other migraine or daily headache medications, such as beta blockers or tricyclics. Administration of fluoxetine with a tricyclic may increase the blood level of the tricyclic compound. Even when fluoxetine does not influence the level of pain, many patients feel that they cope better with the headaches. It is very important to begin with a low dose, 10 mg, and increase to 20 mg if well tolerated. Patients need to be warned about the anxiety, nausea, or insomnia that may occur. Fatigue may be a problem, but is not commonly seen. Fluoxetine is available in 10 and 20 mg capsules and a 20 mg per 5 cc (teaspoon) liquid. For a complete discussion of fluoxetine, see Chapter 3.

Sertraline (Zoloft)

Sertraline is a serotonin reuptake inhibitor, much like fluoxetine. It has only recently been used for migraine or tension headache, but early results are very promising for sertraline's use in both types of headache. Like fluoxetine, sertraline may be utilized in conjunction with tricyclics, but increased tricyclic levels may result. Sertraline has a shorter half-life than that of fluoxetine. The lack of weight gain and sedation are a distinct advantage for sertraline over the older tricyclics, and the anticholinergic side effects are minimal. Sertraline is an effective antidepressant.

Dosage

Sertraline is available in 50 and 100 mg scored tablets. The scored tablets render dosage adjustments very convenient. Adjusting the dose is difficult with fluoxetine because of the capsule. Sertraline is initiated with one half of a 50 mg tablet, increasing to one tablet after 4 days. The dose may then be pushed to 100, 150, or even 200 mg. For depression, the dose varies widely, between 25 and 200 mg per day. Sertraline should be administered once daily, either in the morning or evening. Sertraline is expensive, and it is less costly to work with the 100 mg tablets; one half of a 100 mg tablet is less expensive than one 50 mg tablet.

Side Effects

The side effects of sertraline are similar to those of fluoxetine, with nausea, diarrhea, headache, dry mouth, fatigue, dizziness, tremor, insomnia, sexual dysfunction, constipation, or increased sweating occurring in between 8% and 21% of patients. Anxiety or nervousness may also be a problem. Sertraline is, in general, very well tolerated.

Protriptyline (Vivactil)

This is an extremely valuable medication for prevention of daily headaches because of its lack of sedation. Protriptyline and fluoxetine are two medications for daily headaches that are not usually sedating. Unlike amitriptyline, protriptyline is only occasionally helpful in migraine. Although generally not as effective as amitriptyline, protriptyline has a role in patients where the weight gain or sedation of amitriptyline pose a problem. Combining protriptyline with a beta blocker offsets the tachycardia of protriptyline, and the combination is helpful for patients where both migraine and daily headaches are a problem.

Dosage

The pills are available in 5 and 10 mg tablets, and it is best to start at one half of a 5 mg tablet each morning, slowly increasing to 5 or 10 mg each morning. The doses for depression are usually 20 to 40 mg per day, and the doses for headache are 5 to 30 mg per day. If well tolerated, protryptiline may be pushed to 50 mg per day. Many patients do well on only 5 mg per day. Protriptyline may be combined, in certain circumstances, with a sedating tricyclic at night, such as amitriptyline.

Side Effects

Nervousness, dry mouth, tachycardia, and constipation are common. Dizziness is often seen, as is insomnia. Blurred vision, another anticholinergic side effect seen with both protriptyline and amitriptyline, may occur. Patients may occasionally complain of stomach upset, but protriptyline may be used with ulcer patients. Sedation is rare, and weight gain is extremely uncommon.

Nortriptyline (Pamelor, Aventyl)

This medication is better tolerated than amitriptyline, but somewhat less effective. It is a metabolite of amitriptyline, with essentially the same side effects. However, sedation, dry mouth, constipation, and tachycardia are less severe than with amitriptyline. Nortriptyline is more expensive than amitryptyline.

TABLE 7.4. Tricyclic Antidepressants for Chronic Daily Headache.

Name	A	B	C	D	E	F	G
Amitriptyline								
(Elavil)	4	2	3	2	4	31–46	10–200
Doxepin								
(Sinequan)	2	1	3	2	2	8–24	10–200
Nortriptyline								
(Pamelor, Aventyl)	3	2	2	1	2	18–28	10–200
Protriptyline								
(Vivactil)	3	3	1	1	3	55–124	5–50
Desipramine								
(Norpramin)	3	4	1	1	1	14–62	25–250
Trimipramine								
(Surmontil)	1	1	3	2	2	7–30	25–150

A = blocking of serotonin uptake
B = blocking of norepinephrine uptake
C = sedation
D = orthostatic hypotension
E = anticholinergic
F = half-life, in hours
G = dose range, in mg
1 = small   2 = moderate   3 = high   4 = extremely high

Dosage

As with all antidepressants used for headache, the dose needs to be started at a low level and increased very slowly; 10 mg should be used once each night for 4 nights, then increased to 25 mg at night. The dose may be pushed to 50 mg or more. Many patients do well with as little as 10 or 25 mg, and the side effects are much less at these lower doses. The effective doses for headache tend to be much lower than the effective antidepressant dose. Forms available: Pamelor; 10, 25, 50, and 75 mg capsules and a solution of 10 mg per 5 cc (teaspoon). Aventyl; 10 and 25 mg capsules and a liquid, 10 mg per 5 cc (teaspoon). A generic preparation is now available.

Side Effects

Side effects are very similar to those of amitriptyline, with dry mouth, sedation, weight gain, tachycardia, and constipation being common. However, nortriptyline is better tolerated than amitriptyline, and the anticholinergic side effects are less severe. Nortriptyline is one of the safest tricyclics for older patients with cardiac disease. As with amitriptyline, patients may occasionally experience anxiety or insomnia with nortriptyline, but most patients are less anxious and have improved sleeping with this drug. Nortriptyline is occasionally useful in preventing migraine headaches.

Doxepin (Sinequan)

Doxepin is very similar to amitriptyline in terms of side effects and efficacy. Although doxepin is more effective than nortriptyline in migraine and daily headache, the anticholinergic side effects often limit its usefulness. Sedation, dry mouth, weight gain, and constipation are frequent. Doxepin is only available as a capsule. The dose needs to be initiated with a small amount, 25 mg each night, and gradually increased to 50 or 100 mg. Low doses of 25 to 50 mg are often effective, and as little as 10 mg may help. As with amitriptyline, doxepin at night may be combined with fluoxetine or protriptyline in the morning. Doxepin is available in 10, 25, 50, 75, 100, and 150 mg capsules. (See Chapter 3.)

Desipramine (Norpramin)

Desipramine is a well tolerated antidepressant that is somewhat less effective than the drugs listed above, but is well tolerated. The anticholinergic and sedative side effects are less than with amitriptyline, doxepin, or nortriptyline. Desipramine is not usually effective for migraine prophylaxis, and should only be used for daily headaches.

Dosage

Desipramine is not as effective as amitriptyline, and higher doses are generally necessary. The usual effective dose varies between 50 and 200 mg. Begin with 10 mg each day for 4 days, progress up to 25 mg each day, and then slowly increase to 50 mg. If sedation does not occur with desipramine, the medication may be utilized in the morning. As with any medication, searching for the lowest effective dose is important. Desipramine may be combined with most other migraine preventives, such as amitriptyline at night, or with a beta blocker. The combination of a sedating tricyclic (amitriptyline, doxepin) at night with a nonsedating one (protriptyline, desipramine) in the morning is occasionally the best route to follow. Desipramine is available in 10, 25, 50, 75, 100, and 150 mg tablets.

Side Effects

Side effects are very similar to amitriptyline, but with less anticholinergic effects. Sedation is less than is seen with amitriptyline, but sleep disturbances are more common. Desipramine is frequently best used in the morning because of the sleep disturbance. There is less weight gain with desipramine than with many of the antidepressants, but patients may still gain weight.

Trimipramine (Surmontil)

Trimipramine is a sedating antidepressant that is usually well tolerated. Patients who do not respond to the other antidepressants may occasionally do well with trimipramine. The dosage and side effects are very similar to those of amitriptyline. Trimipramine is worth considering if the patient has responded to amitriptyline but it is no longer effective, or if side effects limit the use of amitriptyline.

Dosage

The usual starting dose is 25 mg, and then we progress to 50 mg over 1 week; the dose may be pushed to 150 mg. The average dose for headache is 50 mg at night. Trimipramine is available in 25, 50, and 100 mg capsules.

Side Effects

Side effects are very similar to those of amitriptyline, with constipation, sedation, dry mouth, and fatigue being common.

Nonsteroidal Anti-inflammatories (NSAIDs)

In older patients, the NSAIDs have limited utility on a daily basis because of the liver, renal, and gastrointestinal side effects. However, in younger patients they may be used if blood tests are performed regularly. The lack of CNS side effects is a major advantage, and the NSAIDs are helpful in patients with concurrent arthritis. Menstrual cramps and menstrual migraines may respond to NSAIDs (see Chapter 4). I often begin utilizing a NSAID as an abortive on an "as needed" basis, and later convert the NSAID to daily use as a preventive medication. For example, if a patient is given amitriptyline as a preventive, and also given Anaprox as an abortive, if the amitriptyline is not tolerated it may be discontinued, and the Anaprox switched to daily use. When patients already possess a medication that they are using as an abortive, it is easy to convert them to daily use of that medication.

The primary NSAIDs that I utilize for CDH include the following: (1) naproxen (Naprosyn, Anaprox), (2) fenoprofen (Nalfon), (3) flurbiprofen (Ansaid), and (4) ketoprofen (Orudis). These medications are extensively discussed in Chapters 2 and 3. Patients may respond to one NSAID and not to another. In younger patients, it often is worthwhile to continue to search for an anti-inflammatory that is effective for that patient.

Miscellaneous NSAIDs

There are many anti-inflammatories that are helpful for daily headaches. The primary NSAIDs utilized for daily headache are listed in the section above. In addition, ibuprofen (Motrin) is well tolerated and helps many patients; it is available over the counter. Diclofenac sodium (Voltaren) is somewhat better tolerated, with fewer GI effects. A newer NSAID, Lodine, has increased prostaglandin activity and has shown early promise in the treatment of migraine and tension headache. Aspirin is helpful for many patients and is very inexpensive for use on a daily basis.

TABLE 7.5. Quick Reference Guide: Second Line CDH Preventive Medication.
1. Valproate acid (Depakote): Effective for daily headache and migraine; the dose varies widely, from 250 to 2,500 mg per day. GI upset and fatigue are common. Weight gain and alopecia may occur. Need to wait at least 4 weeks before abandoning valproate.
2. Beta blockers: Occasionally useful for daily headache, and very effective for migraine. Often combined with tricyclics or anti-inflammatories. Propranolol (Inderal) and nadolol (Corgard) are commonly used. Fatigue, depression, lower GI cramps, and weight gain may occur. Doses are similar to those used for migraine.
3. Muscle relaxants: Safe but only mildly effective; some patients do respond well to these. Fatigue is a prominent side effect. Cyclobenzaprine (Flexeril) is one of the most effective, but may cause severe fatigue. Orphenadrine (Norflex) is effective for some patients. It is best to utilize nonaddicting muscle relaxants.
4. Calcium channel antagonists (Verapamil): Occasionally effective for daily headache as well as migraine and cluster. Verapamil (Calan, Isoptin, Veralan) is the most effective calcium blocker. The SR tablets allow dosing once per day. Constipation and allergic reactions (with a rash) are common. May be combined with tricyclics or anti-inflammatories.

The dosage of the anti-inflammatories for daily headaches varies widely. We want to keep the dose to a minimum and still maintain efficacy. The typical dose of ibuprofen is 400 to 1,600 mg per day; ibuprofen is available in 200, 400, 600, and 800 mg tablets. Voltaren is usually dosed at 75 to 150 mg per day; it is available in 25, 50, and 75 mg tablets. Ansaid is available in 100 mg tablets, and the usual daily dose for headache prophylaxis is one to three pills per day. Orudis is used at 75 to 150 mg per day; it is available in 25, 50, and 75 mg capsules. Aspirin is dosed at two to six pills (325 mg each) per day. The enteric-coated form helps to buffer the stomach. This is inexpensive and available over the counter.

Each of the anti-inflammatories has slightly different properties, which helps to explain why some patients respond to one but not to another. Whichever NSAID is utilized, regular blood tests need to be performed if the drug is to be used every day. The hepatic and renal functions need to be monitored with these blood tests. Patients should be warned to discontinue the drug if GI pain occurs.

Second Line CDH Preventive Medication

Valproate (Depakote)

Depakote has become increasingly useful and popular as a preventive medication for both migraine and CDH. Despite warnings, there have only been several reported fatalities in adults from valproate, and the medication is usually well tolerated. At this point, the antidepressants remain the mainstay of treatment for daily tension headaches, but many patients cannot tolerate even small doses of an antidepressant. Depakote

TABLE 7.6. Prevention Medication: When to Proceed Quickly with Two Preventive Medications at One Time.

1. With most patients, we utilize one prevention medication at a time, in low doses, slowly raising the dose as needed. Most of the patients appreciate this approach, and are perfectly willing to wait for the medication to work.
2. At times, patients may become extremely frustrated with the headaches, and they desire quick results. When these patients suffer from moderate or severe CDH, with bothersome migraines, it is justified to push ahead at a faster rate with a preventive approach. For instance, amitriptyline and verapamil, or amitriptyline and propranolol, may be initiated at the same time. Alternatively, doses may be increased very quickly. The IV DHE repetitive protocol may be utilized, with one or two preventive medications instituted concurrently. The initial amount of preventive medication utilized for a patient depends upon the severity of the headaches and the frustration level of the patient.
3. Patients with new onset of severe headaches, which are usually daily headaches plus migraine, are often extremely upset and frustrated with the pain. In this situation, pushing preventive medication at a faster pace is justified.

is a reasonable alternative for those patients who have daily headaches that are sufficiently severe to require daily medication.

Depakote often requires at least 3 weeks to become effective, and the dose varies widely among patients. Blood tests need to be done, and Depakote is also expensive. The doses and side effects are the same for daily headaches as they are for migraine. For a discussion of Depakote, see Chapter 3. Valproate is available in the following forms: Depakote; sprinkle capsules, 125 mg and tablets, 125, 250, and 500 mg. Depakene; syrup, 250 mg per 5 cc (teaspoon) and capsules, 250 mg.

Beta Blockers

The beta blockers are often very helpful for CDH, and are worth utilizing if antidepressants or NSAIDs have not been effective. Beta blockers are generally less useful for this type of headache than for migraine. Beta blockers are often combined with tricyclics, because the tachycardia of the tricyclics is offset by the bradycardia of the beta blockers. This is an effective combination for both migraine and daily headache. Propranolol (Inderal) plus amitriptyline (Elavil) is a common combination of preventive medication.

The usual beta blockers used for CDH are propranolol and nadolol. The doses are the same as for migraine prophylaxis (see Chapter 3). Although the sedative and cognitive side effects of the beta blockers limit their use, most patients tolerate them fairly well.

Calcium Channel Blockers

Verapamil (Calan, Isoptin, Veralan) is the calcium channel blocker most often utilized for migraine and cluster headache, and it is helpful for some patients with CDH. Verapamil's utility for CDH demonstrates the fact that the line between migraine and daily headache is blurred. Verapamil is usually dosed at 180 to 480 mg per day, utilizing the convenient SR forms of the medication. The average dose is 180 to 240 mg per day. Calan and Isoptin are both available in the 120, 180, and 240 mg tablets. For a discussion of verapamil, see Chapter 3.

Muscle Relaxants

Muscle relaxants help some patients with CDH (Chronic Daily Headache), but they are somewhat disappointing as headache medications. They are generally very safe, and certain patients do very well with them. Sedation limits their use, and some of the medications in this class are habit forming. Muscle relaxants may be used with patients who have ulcer disease. The addition of caffeine may offset fatigue and enhance efficacy.

Cyclobenzaprine (Flexeril)

Cyclobenzaprine occasionally prevents CDH, but sedation limits its use. Most patients can only tolerate it at night, with one-half or one pill being utilized. Cyclobenzaprine is available as a 10 mg tablet, and I start with one half of a tablet at night. If the patient tolerates it well, I slowly increase the close to as much as one pill 3 or 4 times a day. There is a wide range of side effects such as drowsiness, dizziness, lightheadedness, nausea, confusion, dry mouth or anticholinergic problems, and tachycardia or hypotension. Cyclobenzaprine may be combined with anti-inflammatories. Caffeine may help to offset the fatigue.

Orphenadrine Citrate (Norflex)

Norflex is a useful nonaddicting medication that may help to prevent daily headaches. Orphenadrine is an anticholinergic that functions as a muscle relaxant. It does not irritate the stomach, and may be used in patients with GI ulcers. Norflex is available as 100 mg tablets, and is dosed at once or twice per day. The anticholinergic side effects may be disturbing, particularly dry mouth, tachycardia, and blurred vision. Sedation is common, as is lightheadedness. Combining Norflex with acetaminophen in ulcer patients, or with NSAIDs in patients without GI disease, may be helpful. Caffeine may help to offset the fatigue, and increase efficacy.

Methocarbamol (Robaxin)

Generic methocarbamol is an inexpensive muscle relaxant that is well tolerated. It is available in 500 and 750 mg tablets. The usual dose is 500 or 750 mg 1 to 4 times a day. I start with a tiny dose, one half of a 500 mg tablet at night, and slowly increase the dose. As with all muscle relaxants, fatigue, lightheadedness, and dizziness are common. Methocarbamol may be combined with NSAIDs or acetaminophen for an added effect. Caffeine may enhance the efficacy and offset the fatigue.

TABLE 7.7. Quick Reference Guide: Third Line Prevention Therapy for CDH.

1. Polypharmacy: Combinations of two of the first or second line preventives are often very effective. Tricyclics may be combined with NSAIDs or beta blockers; NSAIDs may also be combined with beta blockers or verapamil. Valproate (Depakote) may be combined with tricyclics, beta blockers, or verapamil. The various preventive medications possess different mechanisms of action.
2. MAO inhibitors (phenelzine): Phenelzine (Nardil) is a powerful medication for migraine and daily headache. Use is limited because of dietary restrictions, weight gain, and insomnia. Phenelzine is also effective for depression and anxiety. Combining phenelzine with tricyclics, beta blockers, verapamil, or NSAIDs often enhances the efficacy.
3. Repetitive IV DHE: Four to nine injections of 1 mg DHE are utilized over 2 to 4 days, either in the hospital or, preferably, as an outpatient. More effective for migraine, but daily headache often responds to DHE. DHE is useful in helping to withdraw patients off of analgesics. This is a safe but expensive therapy.
4. Tranquilizers: Occasionally effective for daily headache, but habit forming. Benzodiazepines or phenobarbital are the primary sedatives used for daily headache. Doses need to be minimized, and patients must be carefully monitored.
5. Amphetamines: Helpful for some patients as an "end of the line therapy".

Third Line Prevention Therapy for CDH
(Chronic Daily Headache)

If the above first and second line therapies do not help, there are five avenues open to us: (1) polypharmacy, or combining two of the first or second line medications, (2) MAO inhibitors, such as phenelzine (Nardil), (3) repetitive IV DHE therapy, (4) tranquilizers, and (5) amphetamines.

Polypharmacy

Unlike the situation with epilepsy, polypharmacy increases the effectiveness of headache therapy. We always want to use as little medication as possible, and only resort to polypharmacy if single medications have not been effective. The tricyclics may be combined with NSAIDs or beta blockers, and the NSAIDs may be combined with beta blockers. Depakote may be used with antidepressants or beta blockers, but the combination of Depakote and NSAIDs needs to be monitored very carefully for hepatic irritation. Common combinations of medications include amitriptyline and propranolol, or amitriptyline and Depakote. With increased medication we risk side effects, but we are doing this in patients whose quality of life is severely compromised because of the headaches.

MAO Inhibitors (Phenelzine)

For any of the following medications, patients need to be informed of the side effects, as listed in the PDR and package insert. Phenelzine (Nardil) is a powerful antidepressant that is very effective for both migraine and CDH. Patients on Nardil should be extremely careful about diet and other medications, and the physician needs to trust the patient to be compliant with the restrictions. Being placed on a MAO is a major inconvenience for the patient, as every trip to a restaurant becomes an adventure. Weight gain and insomnia limit the usefulness of Nardil, but for some patients this medication is the only effective treatment for headache. Nardil may be used alone or in combination with tricyclics, beta blockers, or calcium blockers (verapamil). Nardil plus amitriptyline or Nardil plus nortriptyline is a powerful combination for the treatment of daily headache and migraine. Sumatriptan cannot be used with MAOIs. For a full discussion of Nardil therapy, please see Chapter 3.

Repetitive IV DHE Therapy

Repetitive IV DHE (4 to 9 injections of 1 mg) is utilized primarily for migraine and cluster headache. However, many patients with CDH respond well to IV DHE. I have developed a protocol for outpatient repetitive IV DHE in the office, and I feel that four outpatient injections over 2 days provides almost as much relief as the hospital routine. Patients are much more likely to attempt this therapy if they can remain as outpatients, and it is significantly less expensive than hospitalization. The repetitive DHE helps to wean patients off pain medication, and the DHE provides a good start in improving the headache. A preventive medication is initiated while the patient receives the DHE. For a discussion of IV DHE, see Chapter 3.

Tranquilizers

Although not ideal therapy for headache, with certain patients the only effective treatment for CDH lies in the sedative class of medications. If other avenues have been tried, and the patient is able to maintain a low dose, this treatment is justified. For patients with severe daily headaches, a low dose of a benzodiazepine is justified if it is effective. Phenobarbital is effective in some patients, usually at a dose of 60 to 120 mg to night. When I take patients off of daily narcotics or similar analgesics, I often give phenobarbital at night. If the patients then do well with their headaches, it may be worthwhile to continue the phenobarbital. These medications are helpful for those patients whose anxiety is severe and have not responded to relaxation, biofeedback, psychotherapy, or non-addicting medications for anxiety. There are many patients in this category. Patients addicted to the butalbital medications often do well with phenobarbital.

Sample antianxiety agents that are occasionally helpful in CDH include clonazepam (Klonopin), chlordiazepoxide (Librium), and diazepam (Valium). The idea with these is to keep the dose low and limit it per day and per month. Sedation, rebound sleep disturbances, mood swings, depression, and addiction are all hazards of this therapy. These medications do not usually irritate the liver, kidneys, or GI tract.

Clonazepam (Klonopin) is particularly helpful with insomnia, and may be effective for migraine as well as daily headache. Sedation can be severe with clonazepam. The usual dose is 0.5 mg once at night, which may be titrated up to 2 mg total for the day, in split doses. Do not exceed 2 mg for the day. Clonazepam is available in 0.5, 1, and 2 mg tablets.

Chlordiazepoxide (Librium) is an older antianxiety agent that is relatively mild and generally very well tolerated. The usual dose is 5 or 10 mg twice per day, increasing to a maximum of 30 mg (this is a very conservative limit). It is available in capsules of 5, 10, and 25 mg. Chlordiazepoxide is the primary ingredient in Librax, a commonly used medication for irritable bowel.

Diazepam (Valium) is helpful for many conditions. Some patients may find diazepam useful as an abortive for migraine (to induce sleep and relax cervical muscles). For CDH, if other avenues have not been helpful, diazepam may be used if the dose is minimized and the patient understands that it is habit forming. The usual dose is 2 mg twice a day, increasing to 5 mg twice a day if necessary. Do not exceed 10 mg per day on a daily basis. Diazepam is available in 2, 5, and 10 mg tablets.

Amphetamines

As a "last resort," patients may experience less migraine or CDH with Methylphenidate, Dexedrine, or Desoxyn. Insomnia, anxiety, and dependance are possible problems. Doses should be minimized. Doses of Methylphenidate vary from 20 mg to 40 mg per day. Dexedrine is usually dosed at 5 mg or 10 mg BID. Desoxyn is dosed at 2.5 mg or 5 mg BID. Side effects, as listed in the PDR, need to be explained to the patient.

CHAPTER 8

Tension Headache
Sample Case Studies

Sample Case #1: Severe CDH and Occasional Migraine

Joseph is a 48-year-old man with a 13 year history of severe daily headache and a moderate migraine every 2 to 3 months. The migraine headaches do not bother him very much, but the daily headaches are debilitating. They hurt in a band-like distribution about his head, and are often accompanied by moderate to severe neck pain, more on the right. Joseph sleeps well and does not have any medical problems other than the headaches. He is under moderate stress, but states emphatically that stress plays only a minor role in exacerbating his headaches.

Joseph has been refractive to propranolol (Inderal), verapamil (Isoptin, Calan, Veralan), and amitriptyline (Elavil). In the past, he has had periods of time where he overused prescription painkillers such as codeine; he would consume as many as 12 per day. Joe now uses multiple OTC preparations, including six aspirin and caffeine pills, four ibuprofen, and six acetaminophen tablets per day. Relaxation therapy has been mildly beneficial, but Joe does not practice it, as he states that he is too busy and he forgets to do the deep breathing.

With Joe, we need to institute effective prevention medication, decrease or eliminate the analgesics, and encourage him to utilize the relaxation/ deep breathing therapy. As little as 10 or 20 seconds of deep breathing are often sufficient to decrease the intensity of the tension headache; I encourage patients to do this periodically while working or driving.

Joe is experiencing rebound headache, and we need to eliminate this by curtailing the pain medications that he uses throughout the day. After he is off of the pain medications, we will be able to observe the intensity of his daily headaches. Considerations for preventive medication include tricyclic antidepressants, valproate (Depakote), fluoxetine (Prozac), sertraline (Zoloft), or MAO inhibitors (phenelzine). Repetitive IV DHE may also be helpful. Joe has been refractive to amitriptyline, but it may be worth retrying a tricyclic antidepressant.

We decide to begin with protriptyline (Vivactil), an excellent tricyclic for headaches that is not sedating and does not cause weight gain. Since protriptyline often causes a sleep disturbance, patients with insomnia should not be put on this medication. He is given 5 mg tablets of protriptyline (Vivactil) and instructed to take one half of a pill each morning for 4 days, and then to increase it to one tablet each morning. This is a low dose, and may be pushed to 20 or 30 mg, or even higher. As an abortive, we give Joe Norgesic Forte, a nonaddicting combination of aspirin, caffeine, and orphenadrine, and we ask him to limit this to two per day. He is to try one half of a pill at a time, and, if absolutely necessary, to go up to one whole pill. It is crucial with daily headache patients to limit abortive medication. Joe is told to discontinue the OTC medication.

Two weeks later, Joe calls, and he is not improved. We push the protriptyline to 10 mg each morning for 4 days, and then 10 mg twice a day, in the morning and afternoon. On this dose, he does not sleep as well, he has a moderately dry mouth, and he is mildly constipated. We are at the limit of the protriptyline with Joe. He states that his headaches are 30% improved, and he is sticking to the two Norgesic Forte per day, which do help. We want to limit the Norgesic Forte to two per day with Joe. At this point, the decision whether to add more daily preventive medication is a difficult one; we usually attempt to improve the headaches significantly, but not overmedicate the patient. We need to strike a compromise between the head pain and medication, and not try to improve the pain 100%. Much of the decision as to whether to add medication rests on the patient's shoulders and depends on their tolerance for the headaches and for medication.

Joe decides that he truly would like to improve the headaches to a greater degree, and he is willing to change or add medicine. The protriptyline does help, and we would not want to use protriptyline and fluoxetine (Prozac) at the same time. We decide to add valproate (Depakote). Joe is told that it may take 3 weeks for the Depakote to become effective. He is placed on 250 mg of Depakote twice a day, with food. If he tolerates it well, after 1 week Joe is instructed to increase this to 500 mg twice a day. Since we wish to limit aspirin while utilizing Depakote, we switch Joe's abortive to Aspirin Free Excedrin, which is acetaminophen plus caffeine. This is strictly limited to three tablets per day.

What we have done is push one medication, protriptyline, to its limit with this patient. Then, when we are not satisfied with the amount of headache relief, we add another preventive medication. Joe calls 1 week later, and states that he is mildly fatigued on the 250 mg twice a day of Depakote. He has noticed no difference in the headache pattern. We then increase the Depakote to only 750 mg per day, in divided doses. He comes into the office 5 days later for a blood test (because of the

Depakote), and states that he is extremely fatigued, and does not wish to stay with the Depakote. In certain situations, it is important to encourage patients to stick with a medication despite its side effects, particularly when we are on second or third line medicine. With some medications, we know that certain side effects will fade with time. In Joe's situation, however, we decide to discontinue the Depakote. Although Depakote has been a very effective drug for many headache patients, the fatigue, nausea, alopecia, or weight gain may limit its use.

Joe states that he has moderate relief with the protriptyline, 20 mg total per day, and the Aspirin Free Excedrin helps to a small degree. He does not wish to perform the relaxation techniques, as they only help him for 10 minutes.

At this point, we still do not wish to utilize an MAOI, such as phenelzine (Nardil), because of all the problems with the MAOIs. There remain milder alternatives that we could utilize with Joe. We stop the protriptyline and begin fluoxetine (Prozac), 20 mg, one-half capsule each morning for 4 days, then increasing to one capsule each morning. Joe is warned about the possibility of nausea, nervousness, fatigue, or not sleeping as well. His dry mouth and constipation that occured with the protriptyline should resolve with the Prozac. The plan would be to push up the Prozac, if necessary, or add a sedating tricyclic at night, such as doxepin (Sinequan).

Joe calls 2 weeks later and states that he feels better on the Prozac, with mild to moderate headaches, and no side effects other than very mild insomnia. He uses three of the Aspirin Free Excedrin tablets per day. He wishes to improve the headaches, hopefully to a mild level. Joe is instructed to increase the Prozac to two capsules each morning. He calls 1 week later and states that this has helped the headaches, but he cannot sleep. We then back off of the Prozac to one and a half capsules a day, or the 10 mg capsules could be utilized. Joe's headaches increase, and we go back to the two Prozac per day, all in the morning. In Joe's case, we are running out of preventive options, and it may be better to treat the side effect, in this case the insomnia, than to switch medication. In treating his insomnia, we want to utilize a medicine that may further alleviate his headaches. The choices are a sedating tricyclic, such as doxepin, or a benzodiazepine, such as clonazepam (Klonopin). Klonopin is particularly helpful for many headache patients.

Joe is kept on the two Prozac per day and 10 mg of doxepin is added at night. Doxepin is usually as effective as amitriptyline in the treatment of headache. Prozac and the tricyclics, such as doxepin, are useful in combination, and the effects seem additive. This is unlike the situation with depression or epilepsy, where we strive to use monotherapy. Joe states that he sleeps better with the doxepin, but his dry mouth has returned. We instruct him to use the OTC preparations for dry mouth, such as the Biotene products. There are OTC gels, mouthwashes, and toothpastes available for dry mouth. His headaches are 70% improved, and he only uses three pills of Aspirin Free Excedrin on a daily basis. Other considerations for Joe would be increasing Prozac or doxepin, utilizing Klonopin at night, or switching completely to an MAOI, such as phenelzine. The IV DHE protocol, four to nine injections, may help, and this can be done in the office as an outpatient. Under any circumstance, we need to avoid the situation where Joe is consuming vast amounts of analgesics.

Sample Case #2: Moderate to Severe CDH, Plus Anxiety and Depression

Karen is a 26-year-old woman with a 6 year history of moderate to severe CDH, moderate anxiety, and mild to moderate chronic depression. Once every 2 months she has a migraine headache, but Karen does not feel that this is a problem. She has had a small degree of help with biofeedback-relaxation, but she does not like to do the deep breathing, and feels that it is a waste of time. Karen has been in psychotherapy for several years, which helps her depression and anxiety, but not the headaches. Karen feels that a part of her depression is due to the daily headaches. When we diminish the headaches, concomitant depression often improves.

Karen was previously on amitriptyline and nortriptyline, which were too sedating for her. Fluoxetine (Prozac) gave her severe nausea and insomnia. Karen usually sleeps well. The amitriptyline did help her headaches, but the sedation was severe. Benzodiazepines made her more depressed and did not help the headaches.

The idea with Karen would be to find an antidepressant for her headaches that she could tolerate. Logical choices would include desipramine (Norpramin) or protriptyline (Vivactil). Protriptyline may be too "activating" for Karen, thereby increasing her anxiety. Therefore, we institute desipramine, which is a milder, well tolerated tricyclic. I usually begin with 10 mg, a tiny dose, and slowly increase the dose, with the final dose ranging from 25 to 200 mg (or more) per day. Karen is given 10 mg of desipramine to take at night. As an abortive I give Karen naproxen sodium (Anaprox D.S.) to take up to two per day, with food. She has been refractive to all of the OTC preparations. We want to avoid caffeine because of her anxiety.

Karen tolerates 10 mg very well, and we increase the dose, after 4 days, to 25 mg. She has mild insomnia with this. I then change the desipramine to 25 mg each morning. Her headaches are mildly improved after several weeks, and we try to increase the dose further, to 35 mg in the morning, and then to 50 mg each day. Karen feels that the 50 mg dose has decreased her headaches to a moderate level, but she has mild insomnia, dry mouth, and has noticed a tachycardia, partilcularly with exercise. Her resting heart rate is now 92 beats per minute, whereas prior to the desipramine it was 70 beats per minute. We cannot push the dose further, without first instituting a beta blocker. The beta blockers, such as propranolol (Inderal), nadolol (Corgard), or atenolol (Tenormin), decrease headaches and offset the tachycardia of the tricyclic antidepressants. Although a beta blocker may be helpful for Karen's anxiety, it could possibly increase her depression. Patients need to be warned about the possible depression with the beta blockers. Beta blockers do not usually increase depression that is already present; they may, however, initiate a depression.

We keep Karen on the 50 mg of desipramine, and begin atenolol (Tenormin), one half of a 50 mg tablet each night. The usual dose for atenolol is 50 to 100 mg each day. After 1 week, she states that her pulse rate is lower and she can exercise again. The daily headaches remain moderate, and she wishes to try and improve this. At this point, in addition to increasing the desipramine, it may also be helpful to increase the atenolol, because of the tachycardia and the headaches. Increased atenolol may also help her anxiety. We thus increase the desipramine to 75 mg and the atenolol to one whole 50 mg tablet. The plan is to consider increasing the desipramine to 100 mg or more.

Karen does well for 3 months, but then the headaches break through, and she has severe daily headaches again. Her pulse is 80, and we increase the desipramine to 125 mg per day, and then, after 1 week, to 150 mg. She feels very fatigued on this dose, with a severe dry mouth, and we decide to try another preventive approach. The Anaprox did help her previously, but is no longer effective. We substitute Midrin as an abortive. Although Midrin is usually used for migraine, it is often helpful for daily tension headaches as well, and is not addicting. We need to avoid caffeine with Karen, as she has an anxiety disorder, and Midrin does not contain caffeine. Karen does feel that the desipramine has been somewhat helpful for her depression.

We taper Karen off of atenolol and desipramine, as they are no longer effective, and after 1 month we begin phenelzine (Nardil). This MAOI is very effective for daily headaches and migraines, and is also useful for Karen's anxiety and depression. I usually begin phenelzine with one of the 15 mg tablets each night, and slowly increase to three tablets each night. With the MAOIs, using the medication all at night decreases the risk of a hypertensive reaction. (For a complete discussion of phenelzine for headache patients, see Chapter 3.) In carefully selected patients, the MAOIs are usually not a problem. The patients need to be willing to be extremely careful about their diet. I give patients gelcaps of 10 mg Procardia, to cut or bite and put under their tongue if they feel symptoms of a hypertensive reaction.

As an abortive with Karen, I change from Midrin, which cannot be used with phenelzine, to flurbiprofen (Ansaid). Ansaid is often as effective as Anaprox, and Karen had become refractive to the Anaprox.

Karen has mild insomnia from phenelzine, but otherwise tolerates it well. For the insomnia, it is helpful to use the phenelzine in the morning. Her headaches do not decrease until we proceed to three of the Nardil tablets each morning. Ansaid is only mildly helpful for Karen. We do not want to utilize stronger pain medications. It is consistently best if we do not "chase" after the pain all day, but simply try and ignore the milder headaches. With Karen, we change from Ansaid to Anacin, one or two tablets at a time, with a limit of four per day. Excedrin E.S. may be more effective than Anacin, but the extra caffeine in Excedrin may exacerbate Karen's anxiety. Each caffeine in Excedrin may exacerbate Karen's anxiety. Each Anacin tablet contains only 32 mg of caffeine.

Karen does reasonably well on the Nardil and Anacin for several months, but then she complains of weight gain (20 pounds) and insomnia. At this point, Karen's anxiety, depression, and daily headaches are all improved, and we should attempt to decrease the Nardil to two (or even one) pills a day, but keep her on the medication. As an alternative, we could stop the Nardil and use atenolol plus desipramine once again. At times, when a medication has ceased being effective, it may be utilized with success once again at a later date. Other options with Karen are IV DHE therapy in the office or hospital, Valproate (Depakote), or another antidepressant, such as protriptyline (Vivactil). We may want to treat the insomnia with a sedating tricyclic, such as amitriptyline or doxepin, or with a benzodiazepine, such as Klonopin.

CHAPTER 9

Introduction to Cluster Headache and Cluster Headache Abortive Medication

Introduction to Cluster Headache

Cluster headache is among the most severe pains known to mankind. It is characterized by excruciating, debilitating pain lasting from 15 to 180 minutes, and occasionally longer. The pain is usually located around or through one eye, or on the temple. The series of cluster headaches usually lasts several weeks to several months, once or twice per year. Clusters may occur every other year, or even less frequently. Several of the following are usually present: lacrimation, nasal congestion, rhinorrhea, conjunctival injection, ptosis, miosis of the pupil, or forehead and facial sweating. Nausea, bradycardia, and general perspiration also occur in many patients. Attacks usually recur on the same side of the head. Cluster headaches tend to occur more in spring and fall. There is usually no family history of cluster headache, but occasionally there is such a family history.

Specific Characteristics of Cluster Headaches (See Table 9.1)

Males are afflicted more than females, by at least a 6:1 ratio. The onset of the clusters is usually between age 20 and 45, but there are many cases of clusters in teenagers, and occasionally clusters begin in the 50s or 60s, and rarely in the 70s. Approximately one out of 250 men has cluster headaches. Women tend to have an older age of onset for their clusters than men.

The pain of the cluster attack is extreme and starts very quickly, without an aura or a warning. Within minutes, it becomes very severe. Although the pain is usually located about the eye or temple, it may be more intense in the neck or facial areas. Although usually unilateral, the pain does change sides in 10% to 15% of patients, either during a cluster cycle, or the next cycle may see pain on the opposite side. The pain itself is excruciating, described in various manners as sharp, stabbing, "like my eye is being pulled out", and, occasionally, throbbing.

TABLE 9.1. Typical Characteristics of Patients with Cluster Headache.

Begin between ages 20 and 45
Male predominance (6:1)
Same time of year, with no headache in between the cluster cycles
Primarily nocturnal attacks
During cluster cycle, alcohol triggers the headaches
Severe, excruciating, unilateral pain, usually periorbital
Ipsilateral rhinorrhea, lacrimation, conjunctival hyperemia, sweating of the forehead,
  Horner's syndrome

The length of attacks does vary, but 45 minutes is the average. Cluster patients usually experience one or two headaches per day, but this may increase to as many as seven per 24 hours, or decrease to as little as one or two per week. They usually occur around the same time each day, with the time period 9 p.m. to 10 a.m. being most frequent. Approximately half of the patients awaken from sleep with the headaches.

Cluster cycles, except in the chronic variety, usually last 3 to 8 weeks, and then stop until the next bout of the clusters. The clusters occasionally last as little as several days, or as long as 5 months, at which time we begin to think that they may have converted to the chronic cluster type. Ten percent of cluster patients have chronic clusters, where there is no break of at least 6 months between attacks. One or two bouts of the clusters per year is average for most patients. They may increase in frequency, with only several months in between bouts, or several years may elapse between attacks. When periodic clusters begin at older ages, the chance of conversion to chronic cluster becomes greater. The natural history of clusters is not known, but the tendency is for the cluster series to stop at a certain age. Many patients "lose" their clusters in the late 30s or 40s.

During the cluster series, over half of the patients are very sensitive to alcohol, and most patients will have an attack triggered by ingestion of alcohol. The other "headache" foods are less important, but avoiding MSG, aged cheeses and meats, and chocolate is prudent during the cluster series. MSG, in particular, seems to trigger a more severe cluster in some patients. Cluster patients may have their clusters after stress is over, and occasionally excessive cold, heat, or bright light have been associated with the precipitation of a cluster. However, most cluster patients have very little control over the clusters, except with medication.

The typical episodic cluster series builds over 1 to 2 weeks and peaks for 1 to 3 weeks, and then decreases. In the 10% of cluster patients with chronic clusters, periods of peaks and valleys with the headaches also occur, but the extended break without any clusters is not present. Chronic clusters are not usually consistent throughout the year, but tend to increase in certain seasons. In managing the clusters, we keep in mind the fact that the clusters build and then peak, and I often treat them with somewhat less medication, particularly corticosteroids, in the beginning of a cluster period.

Nonmedication Treatment of Cluster Headache

Other than medication, very little is available for sufferers of cluster headache. The pain is too severe for relaxation methods, and some patients state that biofeedback or relaxation may actually precipitate or increase a cluster. However, learning simple deep breathing techniques or relaxation methods does aid some patients in helping to curb the anticipation of the cluster attacks. Much anxiety is generated during the day when the patient knows that nighttime brings intense, excruciating pain.

Ice to the area of the pain may help, although sometimes heat will be more effective. Some patients let the shower run hot water on their cervical area, or they use a shower water massage apparatus to allow the hot water to run over their cervical or frontal area. Pressing over the temporal area with moderate pressure is occasionally helpful. Cluster patients usually feel better when moving about during an attack.

Medications for Cluster Headache

For most patients, both abortive and preventive medications are helpful, and only in a minority of situations do we simply use abortive medicines. This chapter will focus on the abortive medications, and the following chapter will delve into the preventive approach.

Abortive Medications for Cluster Headache

The abortive treatment of clusters is the same for episodic and for chronic cluster headaches. Since the headache is very intense from the beginning, and the pain is severe and excruciating, medication to aid the attack must act quickly. Most cluster attacks last less than 1 hour, averaging about 45 minutes, and thus oral pain medication is only of limited value. However, in patients whose attacks do last for more than 1 hour, pain medications may be useful, particularly if the standard cluster abortives are not completely effective. Antiemetics are also used for those patients with nausea, and the sedative effect of these is often helpful.

The first line abortive cluster medications are as follows: (1) inhaled oxygen, (2) ergotamine tartrate, (3) sumatriptan injections, and (4) dihydroergotamine (DHE) injections. Second line therapies include: injectable or oral pain medications, intranasal lidocaine, injections of ketorolac (Toradol), and antiemetics, either orally or as suppositories.

TABLE 9.2. Quick Reference Guide: First Line Abortive Medications for Cluster Headache.

1. Oxygen: Very effective, with no side effects. May be combined with other abortives. Oxygen is worth trying for all patients willing to rent a tank; the usual dose is 8 liters/min., with a mask, used sitting up and leaning slightly forward.
2. Ergotamine tartrate: Moderately effective, but with many side effects. Ergostat is a pure ergotamine pill to be used sublingually, and may also be swallowed. Cafergot adds caffeine to the ergotamine. Cafergot PB suppositories are very effective. Side effects of the ergots include anxiety and nausea, both of which may be severe. The rebound headache situation does not usually occur in cluster patients using ergots.
3. Sumatriptan: A very effective cluster and migraine abortive medication. The injections are utilized more extensively for clusters than are the pills. The subcutaneous injections are 6 mg each, with two injections per day being the maximum. Taste disturbances, nausea, tingling or hot sensations, feelings of pressure, chest discomfort, and drowsiness may occur. Oxygen may be utilized simultaneously, along with ice on the site of the cluster pain. Very expensive but effective.
4. Dihydroergotamine (DHE): Similar to sumatriptan, DHE is primarily utilized as an injecton. Nausea, leg cramps, heat flashes, and tightness in muscles may occur. The usual dose is 1 mg IM that may be repeated once, if necessary. DHE is usually somewhat more effective than the standard ergotamines, with fewer side effects.

First Line Cluster Abortive Medications

Oxygen

Oxygen is effective in approximately 80% of cluster headache patients. To obtain a small tank with a mask is relatively easy and not terribly expensive. The tanks are usually rented for 1 month. If feasible, most patients with cluster headaches should attempt to use oxygen for their attacks. The patient should be sitting with the body leaning slightly forward. A mask is used, and 100% oxygen is inhaled at 8 liters per minute. In healthy patients with no pulmonary problems, the oxygen may be inhaled for 1 or 2 hours. They should not utilize more than 2 hours in 1 day. Most patients only use the oxygen for 15 or 20 minutes. A typical small oxygen tank will provide only 3 hours of oxygen at 8 liters per minute. Ice and cluster abortive medications may be combined with the oxygen.

Ergotamine Tartrate

Strong vasoconstrictors, the ergotamines have many limitations, but should be utilized at some point in the treatment of most of the younger cluster patients. Ease of administration (they are available as tablets) is a major advantage for the ergots. The frequent side effects of nausea and nervousness limit their use. In older patients, the risk of angina or an actual myocardial infarction restricts use. The rebound headaches that occur in migraineurs do not seem to be a problem in cluster headache patients. The primary ergotamine preparations are Cafergot pills and suppositories and Ergostat sublingual pills. Peripheral vascular disease or hypertension are contraindications. Ergotamines may exacerbate peptic ulcer disease. The effective dose of ergotamine varies widely among patients. Ergots may be combined with the use of oxygen and other abortive measures.

The most commonly used "standard" ergots, not including DHE, are Ergostat sublingual pills, Cafergot pills, Cafergot suppositories, and Cafergot PB suppositories.

Ergostat Pills

These contain 2 mg of ergotamine tartrate with no caffeine. The usual dose is one pill sublingually at the onset of the cluster attack. Ergostat may also be swallowed, and this route may be just as effective as the sublingual method. This may be repeated once in 1 or more hours, limited to 2 pills per 24 hours.

Nausea is common, as is a bitter or "bad" taste in the mouth. Nervousness is a frequent side effect, but less so than with Cafergot, because there is no caffeine in Ergostat. Ergotamines need to be used with great caution in the presence of hypertension, peripheral vascular disease, or peptic ulcer disease. Unless ergots have been demonstrated to be safe in a patient, it is prudent to first try other medications in patients over the age of 40.

Cafergot Pills

Cafergot consists of 1 mg of ergotamine tartrate and 100 mg of caffeine. Cafergot pills are the most convenient, but least effective, of the ergots.

Dosage is one or two pills at the onset of headache, repeated every $\frac{1}{2}$ hour as needed, with a maximum of five per day and 10 per week. Side effects are similar to the preceding Ergostat discussion, with nausea and nervousness being common. Anxiety or nervousness is more common with Cafergot pills than with Ergostat, because of the caffeine. The same precautions discussed above in the Ergostat section apply to Cafergot.

Cafergot Suppositories

These are less convenient but much more effective than the pills. Cafergot suppositories contain 2 mg of ergotamine tartrate and 100 mg of caffeine. The primary side effects are nausea and anxiety. The Cafergot PB suppositories (see next section) cause much less nausea and are more effective, but this preparation is not always available.

The usual dosage is one third or one half of a suppository, and the dose is then titrated up or down, depending on the patient's response. The effective dose varies widely among patients. The dose may be repeated after 1 hour, up to a maximum of two suppositories per day and five per week. Some patients find that as little as one fifth of a suppository is all that they require.

Side effects of Cafergot suppositories are the same as those of Cafergot pills. Nausea and anxiety always are limiting factors in the use of ergots.

Cafergot PB Suppositories

Similar but more effective than plain Cafergot suppositories, Cafergot PB contains 2 mg of ergotamine tartrate, 100 mg of caffeine, 60 mg of sodium pentobarbital, and 0.25 mg of l-alkaloids of belladonna. Availability of this preparation is a major problem, and at present we often have them made by a compounding pharmacist. The generic preparation is available on a limited basis.

Dosage is the same as for the plain Cafergot suppositories. Side effects are decreased, with less nausea and nervousness. Sedation may be a problem, however.

Sumatriptan Injections

Injectable sumatriptan and DHE are generally more effective therapies than the standard ergots, such as Ergostat or Cafergot. Pills of sumatriptan are more helpful for migraine than for cluster headache. Many patients are reluctant to give themselves injections, but for those who are willing, sumatriptan and DHE are usually effective, with a minimum of side effects. The high cost of sumatriptan will be a limiting factor in its use.

The dosage of sumatriptan is usually 6 mg, given subcutaneously at the onset of the cluster headache. A repeat dose may be given at least 1 hour after the first injection. Two injections, or 12 mg, is the maximum recommended dosage per 24 hours. Sumatriptan is administered subcutaneously by the use of a convenient auto-injector device. If an ergotamine preparation has been taken, 24 hours should elapse prior to using sumatriptan. Following sumatriptan administration, patients need to wait at least 6 hours before using an ergotamine compound.

Daily use of sumatriptan has not been studied extensively, and we do not know how safe daily utilization of sumatriptan is. Thus, until further studies are known, prudent use of sumatriptan would dictate that no more than six injections per week be taken for cluster headache, and less for migraine. For chronic cluster headache, if sumatriptan is used for more than 1 or 2 months, we would have to limit use even further. We need to have more information before we allow patients to use sumatriptan on a daily basis for extended periods, or before we can allow patients to use more than two injections per day.

Oxygen may be used in conjunction with sumatriptan, and escape pain medication may also be utilized. The side effects of sumatriptan are generally less than with DHE. Transient pain at the site of injection is common, and "icing" the injection site prior to use may decrease this burning pain. Other side effects that occur include tingling sensations, disturbances of taste, heat flashes, and feelings of pressure or heaviness. Side effects tend to be short lasting. The pressure feelings may occur in any part of the body. Chest symptoms, flushing, dizziness, and overall weakness may also occur. Minor transient increases in blood pressure have been seen. Nausea is relatively common, but generally less than is seen with DHE. Drowsiness may occur. Sumatriptan should not be used in children or adolescents, in pregnant women, in women who are nursing, in the face of hepatic or renal impairment, or with cardiovascular disease. Patients over the age of 45 should be screened for cardiac risk factors, and sumatriptan has not been approved for use after age 65. The frequent chest pressure that occurs is not usually felt to be of cardiac origin.

DHE

This compound is different from the other ergots in that it is only a mild arterial constrictor; DHE most likely works through serotonergic effects (it is a venoconstrictor). I consider DHE to be safer than the other ergotamines, and I will use DHE in older age ranges if there are no contraindications.

DHE is not effective orally, and is usually given as an IM injection. I have been using DHE as a nasal spray, but this preparation is not yet commercially available, and we need to have it compounded by a pharmacist. For patients willing to give themselves an injection, IM DHE is an extremely effective abortive medication. (For a complete discussion of DHE, see Chapters 2 and 3.)

Second Line Cluster Abortive Medications

These include pain medications, intranasal lidocaine, injectable (IM) ketorolac (Toradol), and antiemetics.

When the first line therapies do not work, I usually give pain medications. In addition, intranasal lidocaine, although generally not very effective, does help some patients. IM ketorolac is helpful at times, and the antiemetics sedate the patient and decrease any associated nausea. Cluster patients become very desperate, and they need to have available any abortive treatment that will offer relief.

Abortive Analgesics for Cluster Headache

The abortive pain medications include the following: Extra-Strength Excedrin, naproxen (Anaprox D.S.), Norgesic Forte, butalbital compounds (Fiorinal or Esgic), and narcotics. These are all discussed in the chapter on abortive medications for migraine (Chapter 2).

In general, we do not want to have cluster patients become addicted to narcotics. The use of injectable narcotics should be monitored and

---

TABLE 9.3. Quick Reference Guide: Second Line Abortive Cluster Headache Medications.

---

1. Analgesics: Pain medications are useful to have available for cluster patients if the first line medications are not very helpful. Psychologically, it is useful for the patient to know that there is at least something available that may ease the pain, even if it is minimal relief. The aspirin containing compounds, such as Excedrin or Norgesic Forte, are occasionally helpful. Naproxen or other anti-inflammatories are sometimes partially effective. Butalbital compounds, such as Fiorinal or Esgic, help to some degree, and are mildly sedating. The narcotics help ease the pain to an extent, but they need to be monitored very carefully. Cluster patients may tend to overuse narcotics because of the extreme intensity of the pain.

2. Intranasal lidocaine: Although not usually very effective, some patients obtain limited relief from 4% intranasal lidocaine. This is administered via a plastic spray bottle, or may be used with a dropper. Lidocaine is a safe adjunctive abortive agent for the clusters, with minimal side effects. It is easy to use, and is worthwhile if it provides even 20% relief for the patient.

3. Ketorolac (Toradol) IM injections: Ketorolac is an anti-inflammatory that is effective for some patients with migraine or cluster headache. It acts rapidly and may be self-administered. Ketorolac may cause GI pain or upset, but is not addicting or sedating. First line medications may be utilized with the ketorolac injection.

4. Antiemetics: Cluster patient may experience nausea, and the antinausea agents are sedating, which helps the patient in tolerating the cluster. Phenergan is very safe, and has a low incidence of side effects other than sedation. Tigan is very well tolerated. Compazine is somewhat more effective, with a higher incidence of adverse reactions, such as anxiety. Chlorpromazine (Thorazine) is a powerful, sedating antiemetic that is helpful for the patient in severe pain; extreme sedation may last up to 24 hours, however.

---

limited. However, in some patients, the pain is so severe, and the first line therapies are not effective, and thus the use of narcotics is justified. The milder approaches, such as Excedrin, should be utilized first, and then the butalbital compounds, and finally the narcotics.

Intranasal Lidocaine for Cluster Headache

Lidocaine spray, as a 4% lidocaine solution, has been used since the mid-1980s for cluster headache. I have found it only mildly effective for most patients, and almost never adequate by itself. However, intranasal lidocaine does provide sufficient relief to warrant its use. The lidocaine is very safe, with minimal side effects. When used in conjunction with ice and one of the other first line abortives, the lidocaine spray can add 10% to 30% relief.

I put 4% topical lidocaine in a plastic nasal spray bottle. The patient is then instructed to lie in the supine position, extend their head back 30 to 45 degrees, turn the head toward the side of the pain, and spray 2 or 3 sprays of the lidocaine intranasally. This may be repeated, but I usually limit the lidocaine sprays to six or eight in a 24 hour period. If the nasal passage is blocked, several drops of 0.5% phenylephrine may be used prior to the lidocaine.

Alternatively to the spray bottle, 1 ml of 4% topical lidocaine may be slowly dropped, via a dropper, into the nostril on the side of the pain. Side effects are minimal. Numbness in the throat may occur, but this is transient. Nervousness or tachycardia occur at times, but are rare.

Injectable Ketorolac (Toradol)

Ketorolac is useful as an abortive, particularly when oral medication cannot be tolerated. It is well tolerated, and patients can learn to self-administer the injections at home. Ketorolac is effective for some cluster patients, has a fast onset of action, and the lack of sedation is very helpful. Ketorolac is not addicting. The ketorolac injections are expensive (approximately ten dollars per injection), but they are conveniently packaged in a single injection unit, and the patient does not have to mix medication from a vial.

Ketorolac is available as a 30 mg per cc injection, or as 60 mg per 2 cc in the prefilled syringes. The usual dose is 60 mg that may then be repeated with another 30 to 60 mg in $\frac{1}{2}$ or 1 hour, if necessary. I limit the injections to once per day for clusters if patients are using it on a daily basis. When used daily, ketorolac should only be utilized for limited periods of time.

GI upset or pain occur frequently, as ketorolac is a nonsteroidal anti-inflammatory. Sedation is infrequent but may occur. Hepatic and renal functions need to be monitored, and ketorolac should not be given in the presence of hepatic or renal impairment.

Antiemetics

A minority of cluster patients experience moderate or severe nausea with their headaches, and treating this is helpful. In addition, the antiemetics are usually sedating, and this can be useful for the cluster patient who is experiencing very severe pain. Promethazine (Phenergan) is a sedating antiemetic with a very low incidence of side effects. Used as a pill or as a suppository, promethazine also potentiates the analgesics. The stronger antiemetics, particularly prochlorperazine (Compazine) and chlorpromazine (Thorazine), also are valuable in some cluster patients. For instance, if nothing is working for a severe cluster attack, a 100 mg suppository of Thorazine will often sedate the patient. For both very severe migraine and cluster headaches, Thorazine may, at times, help the patient to avoid the emergency room. Please refer to Chapter 2 for a complete discussion of antiemetics.

CHAPTER *10*

Cluster Headache Preventive Medication

Most patients with cluster headache require daily prophylactic medication because the headaches are extremely severe and difficult to abort. Some patients experience milder cluster headaches, and if oxygen or another abortive is effective, preventive medications may be avoided. The number of headaches per day is also a determining factor, for if patients have only one per day, we may be able to avoid prevention medication. Cluster sufferers, in general, desire to be on preventive medication during the cluster cycle.

With episodic cluster headache, we utilize medication only when the headaches begin, as it is not worthwhile to keep patients on medication all year for intermittent headaches. For chronic cluster headache, most patients are on continuous daily medication to prevent the clusters. The prophylactic medications for episodic and chronic cluster headaches differ slightly.

Preventive Medication for Episodic Cluster Headache

Cluster headaches often build in intensity over days or weeks. At first, patients may simply feel twinges of pain on the affected side, and then the intensity slowly builds. Usually, the patients will call or visit the physician 1 week or more into the cluster cycle. Once we believe that the cluster cycle has begun, preventive medication should be instituted. Cortisone is the fastest acting medication, and we begin with limited amounts of it. Concurrently, the patient is given another first line prevention medication, either lithium or verapamil. When we have withdrawn the cortisone, the second preventive medication will hopefully have become effective.

The preventive medication is discontinued when the cluster series has finished. If a patient usually experiences a 4 week cycle of clusters, and the current series has lasted 5 weeks with no headache for 1 week, preventive medication may be withdrawn. I wait for the clusters to be

TABLE 10.1. Criteria for the Use of Prevention Medication.

1. The clusters are not easily stopped with abortive medication.
2. Cluster headaches are daily and last longer than 15 minutes.
3. The patient is willing to take daily medication, and endure possible side effects.

TABLE 10.2. Quick Reference Guide: First Line Cluster Preventive Medication.

1. Cortisone: Very effective for cluster headache; is used primarily for episodic clusters. It is given for 1 or 2 weeks during the peak of the cluster series. Prednisone, Decadron, or injectible forms may be utilized. When used for short periods of time, side effects are minimal. A typical regimen is prednisone (20 mg) or Decadron (4 mg) once a day for 3 days, then one-half pill per day for 10 days, then stop. Additional cortisone may be given later in the cycle, when the clusters increase.
2. Verapamil (Calan, Isoptin, Veralan): A well tolerated calcium channel blocker; effective in episodic and chronic cluster. One 240 mg SR pill is taken once or twice per day. This is often initiated at the onset of the headaches, in conjunction with cortisone. Verapamil is then continued after the cortisone is stopped. Constipation is common. Because of its efficacy and a lack of side effects, verapamil is a mainstay of cluster prevention.
3. Lithium: Very helpful for chronic cluster and, to a lesser degree, episodic cluster. Small doses, one to three of the 300 mg tablets per day, are used for cluster headache. May be combined with verapamil and/or cortisone. Lithium is usually well tolerated in low doses; drowsiness, mood swings, nausea, tremor, and diarrhea may occur. Blood tests need to be done.

---

gone for 1 or 2 weeks prior to stopping medication. Patients are instructed to quickly reinstitute the preventive medication if the clusters reappear. A cluster series may drag on for extra weeks or months, well beyond what the patient normally experiences.

First line preventive approaches for episodic cluster include: cortisone, verapamil, lithium, and polypharmacy (combining two first line medications).

Second line preventive medications include: methysergide (Sansert), valproate (Depakote), daily ergotamines, ergonovine, and steroid blockade of the occipital nerve.

Third line preventive medications include: IV dihydroergotamine (DHE) given repetitively, and cocaine drops used intranasally on a daily basis.

Miscellaneous therapies that are occasionally helpful for episodic clusters include: indomethacin (Indocin), phenelzine (Nardil), cyproheptadine (Periactin), nifedipine (Procardia), and beta blockers such as propranolol (Inderal).

Once a regimen is determined effective for a patient, the appropriate medications are instituted at the onset of the next cluster series. Many of the medications used for cluster headache have not received specific FDA indications for this use. The following is only a guide to what I consider reasonable and rational therapy for cluster headeache. Prior to prescribing medications for the patient, the person needs to be informed of, and accept, the complete set of contraindications and side effects as listed in the PDR and package insert.

First Line Preventive Medication for Episodic Clusters

These include cortisone, verapamil, lithium, or a combination of the above. Cortisone has a quick onset of action, but we always want to minimize the dose. When the headaches are not severe, I reserve cortisone for use during the peak time of the clusters. Verapamil and lithium, although excellent cluster headache medications, often take days or weeks to become effective.

Cortisone

We want to use cortisone in the least possible effective dose. I utilize cortisone for only 1 or 2 weeks, and later it may be given again for a period of very severe clusters. Prednisone, dexamethasone (Decadron), or triamcinolone (Aristocort) may be used. At times, one form will work more effectively than another. As injections, ACTH gel and Depo-Medrol usually provide quick relief, with the effect lasting days to 1 week (usually not longer).

I usually utilize 4 mg tablets of Decadron once or twice per day for 3 days, then one-half tablet once or twice per day for 7 to 10 days, then stop. Alternatively, prednisone may be used, 20 mg once or twice per day for 3 days, then 10 mg once or twice per day for 7 to 10 days, then stop. Cortisone should be taken with food. These are relatively low doses. For patients in the midst of a severe cluster cycle, ACTH gel, 60 units, or Depo-Medrol, 60 mg, may be given, and then the oral cortisone is given. Later in the cycle, small amounts of cortisone may be repeated.

Side effects of cortisone are many, but used for short periods of time in low doses, we usually avoid these effects. Many patients become nervous or moody with cortisone, and sleeping problems may occur.

TABLE 10.3. Equivalent Doses of the Glucocorticoids.

Medication	Salt Retention (mineralocorticoid potency)	Dose (app. equiv.) in mg.	Half-life (hours)
Hydrocortisone	High	20	8–12
Prednisone	Medium	5	18–36
Methylprednisolone	None	4	18–36
Triamcinolone	None	4	18–36
Betamethasone	None	0.6–0.75	36–54
Dexamethasone	None	0.75	36–54

The anti-inflammatory strength of dexamethasone and betamethasone is very powerful, with an approximate ratio of 25 for these versus 4 for prednisone, and only 1 for hydrocortisone.

Fluid retention or fatigue may be a problem. GI upset and pain are common. By utilizing smaller doses for short periods of time, we avoid the devastating longer term side effects of the corticosteroids.

Verapamil

Verapamil (Isoptin, Calan, Veralan) is a calcium channel blocker that is very effective in cluster headache and migraine. The lack of major side effects is a distinct advantage. There is very little of the weight gain or lethargy often experienced with other medications. Verapamil may be used with cortisone or Lithium, or simply as a single preventive. Although verapamil may take weeks to become effective, it often takes effect in days. The long acting form (Isoptin SR or Calan SR) is very convenient, with the tablets being scored. The "regular" verapamil pills, not the long acting, may be more effective than the long acting preparation.

Verapamil is usually started early in the cluster cycle, and if the headaches are severe, cortisone may be used in conjunction with the verapamil. Doses are initiated at one half of a 180 or 240 mg SR tablet once per day, quickly increasing to a full tablet. Occasionally, we progress to 480 mg per day, checking for hypotension. The average dose is 240 to 360 mg per day.

Verapamil is generally very well tolerated. Constipation is common, with allergic reactions (rashes), dizziness, insomnia, and anxiety occurring at times. Verapamil may exacerbate or cause chronic daily headache. Fatigue is less common than with the beta blockers, but is seen in some patients. Peripheral edema may occur.

Lithium

Although lithium carbonate is probably more effective for chronic cluster headache, it is helpful for many episodic cluster patients. Low doses, usually one to three of the 300 mg pills, are usually utilized with cluster patients. With low doses, lithium is generally well tolerated. Lithium may be combined with verapamil and/or cortisone. After verapamil and cortisone, lithium is often the next choice for cluster prevention.

I usually begin with one of the lithium carbonate pills, 300 mg, with food, once per day. The patient takes the lithium several hours prior to the expected time of the headache. After several days, the lithium is increased to one 300 mg tablet twice per day; this is the average dose. The tablets may be cut in half, and there are 150 mg capsules of lithium carbonate available. Slow release tablets are available, as is a controlled release tablet (Eskalith CR). Since we usually use low doses of lithium, toxicity is rarely a problem. The lithium may be combined with verapamil, cortisone, or another cluster preventive, if necessary. Occasionally, I will push the lithium to 1,200 or 1,500 mg per day, and monitor serum levels. Blood tests need to be checked with the lithium, and the level monitored, but the clinical effect for cluster headaches does not correlate with the level. The usual serum levels for bipolar illness are 0.6 to 1.2 mEq/l. Toxic doses are close to therapeutic.

Side effects with lithium are many; however, with the small doses utilized for clusters, most patients tolerate the drug very well. Drowsiness, tremor, and mood swings may occur. Diarrhea, nausea, or vomiting may be present. Polyuria and mild thirst are common, particularly in the first week of lithium therapy. Early symptoms of lithium toxicity include vomiting, fatigue, diarrhea, and muscular weakness. Ataxia, blurred vision, and tinnitus usually do not occur unless a more serious toxicity is present.

With long term treatment, hypothyroidism may be a problem. Toxicity is seen with greater frequency in the elderly. Renal and cardiovascular disease preclude the use of lithium. I usually avoid the concomitant use of NSAIDs or diuretics with lithium. By using low doses, with close monitoring, we rarely encounter serious problems with the use of lithium for cluster headaches.

Polypharmacy

As with migraine, the different mechanisms of action of the cluster medications are additive. If one medication is not completely effective, we will use a combination of verapamil, lithium, and cortisone. Lithium with verapamil is a common combination for clusters, and short bursts of cortisone may be utilized.

Second Line Preventive Medication for Episodic Clusters

If the first line medications are not effective, we need to progress to second line therapy, which includes the following: (1) methysergide (Sansert), (2) valproate (Depakote), (3) daily ergotamines, (4) ergonovine, and (5) steroid blockade of the occipital nerve.

Methysergide (Sansert)

Methysergide is much more effective for episodic cluster headaches than for chronic clusters. Because of the possiblility of fibrosis, this drug has declined in popularity, but with judicious use it is a relatively safe and effective medication. The advantage with episodic clusters is that we do not need to use methysergide for extended periods of time. Side effects often limit the use of methysergide, such as the frequent nausea and GI upset. However, for many cluster patients, methysergide will be effective when the first line medications do not help. Methysergide may be combined with other cluster preventives.

Methysergide should be initiated with one pill (the only pill available is 2 mg) per day, with food. I have used as little as one-half pill per day, but

TABLE 10.4. Quick Reference Guide: Second Line Cluster Prevention Medication.

1. Methysergide (Sansert): Effective for episodic clusters, but with many side effects. Nausea, leg cramps, and dizziness are common. Dosage is one to four pills per day, with food; try to attain the least possible dose. The fibrosis issue is not usually a problem with the limited time methysergide is given for episodic clusters.
2. Valproate (Depakote): This seizure medication is becoming increasingly popular for cluster, migraine, and tension headache. Liver functions need to be monitored in the beginning. Useful in both chronic and episodic clusters. Common side effects include lethargy, GI upset, mood swings, weight gain, and alopecia. Dosage ranges from 250 to 2,000 mg per day, in divided doses. The average dose is 1,000 mg per day.
3. Ergotamines (Daily): The rebound situation does not apply with cluster headache. Cafergot, Ergostat SL, or Bellergal-S may be used, usually given several hours prior to the peak time of the clusters. Nausea and nervousness are common with the ergotamines. The lowest effective dose should be utilized.
4. Ergonovine (Ergotrate): Ergotrate is available commercially, or compounding pharmacists prepare the ergonovine. A well tolerated ergotamine derivative, ergonovine is usually dosed at 0.2 mg 2 to 3 times per day. GI upset and anxiety may occur.
5. Steroid blockade of the occipital nerve: By placing cortisone in the region of the occipital nerve, we may provide days to weeks of decreased cluster headache. Depo-Medrol or betamethasone may be used, with a small (25 gauge) needle. Well tolerated, with few side effects. These should be limited to 2 injections per cluster series, at most.

they are difficult to cut in half. The average dose is one pill twice per day. Although higher doses are occasionally more effective, it is best to limit methysergide to four pills per day.

Nausea, occasionally severe, is common, as is a "hot" feeling in the head, and leg cramps. Dizziness is common. Some patients complain of feeling strange on methysergide. These reactions may be severe, and if the patients are warned about them, they will not panic when the extreme side effects do occur. If the side effects are mild, they will often cease if the patient continues for several more days with the drug. Sansert may exacerbate ulcer disease. Contraindications include active peptic ulcers, peripheral vascular disease, cardiac valve problems, or coronary artery disease. Methysergide should be used with caution in patients with hypertension. Methysergide should also be avoided with pregnancy, renal insufficiency, or liver disease.

The rare fibrosis that has been reported is generally not an issue when methysergide is used for episodic clusters, as we only need to utilize the medication for 1 or 2 months. For a complete discussion of the fibrosis, see the section on methysergide in Chapter 3.

Valproate (Depakote)

This medication is usually used for seizures, but has also been very helpful for headache prevention. Depakote has proven useful for migraine, chronic daily, and cluster headache. Valproate needs to be monitored, but it has proven to be a safe and effective medication. Valproate is usually instituted as a second line cluster medication, and has been useful in both episodic and chronic clusters. I usually utilize valproate after lithium, verapamil, cortisone, and Sansert. There is often a delayed onset of action with this medication. However, in treating chronic clusters, this is not as much of a concern as it is with episodic cluster headaches.

I usually begin with low doses of Depakote (the coated tablets of valproate). One 250 mg tablet is taken twice per day, with food, and this may be increased to 1,000 mg per day. If the clusters do not respond, Depakote may be pushed to 2,000 mg per day, in 2 or 3 divided doses. Levels need to be checked for toxicity. Some patients do well on small doses, sometimes as little as 250 or 500 mg per day.

Depakote is fairly well tolerated but nausea, gastritis, sedation, and emotional upset (depression or mood swings) are relatively frequent. Over months to 1 year, weight gain is common. Hair loss, rash, and dose-related tremor also occur. Elevated serum ammonia levels may be seen. Liver functions and blood counts need to be monitored closely in the first several months, but for episodic clusters the entire duration of use is only 1 or 2 months. See Chapter 3 for a complete discussion of valproate.

Ergotamines Taken Daily

Although we usually wish to avoid daily ergots in headache patients, the rebound headache situation encountered by migraine patients does not usually occur with cluster sufferers. The medication is typically utilized for only 4 to 8 weeks, and once the cluster episode is over, the ergots may easily be discontinued.

I attempt to time the use of ergotamines to be given within several hours of the expected cluster attack. If the headache typically occurs at 11 p.m. The patient takes the ergotamine at 9 or 10 p.m. The usual dose is 1 or 2 mg per day, and this may be increased to 4 mg per day.

Cafergot may be used as the source of ergotamine, but the caffeine increases side effects. Cafergot pills contain 1 mg of ergotamine and 100 mg of caffeine. The suppositories contain 2 mg of ergotamine and 100 mg of caffeine. The Cafergot preparations are more useful earlier in the day.

Ergostat sublingual pills contain 2 mg of ergotamine and no caffeine. These may be ingested at night without the associated insomnia of the Cafergot. I instruct patients to swallow the pills.

Bellergal-S is a compound that contains 0.6 mg of ergotamine, 40 mg of phenobarbital, and 0.2 mg of belladonna. The sedation of phenobarbital is occasionally helpful for the cluster patient. However, the 0.6 mg of ergotamine is usually insufficient to prevent the cluster attack.

The usual side effects of ergotamines are nausea and nervousness. Many patients cannot tolerate ergots, and I use the ergotamine compounds with great caution after age 40 or 45. For a complete discussion of ergotamines, please see Chapter 2.

Ergonovine

Ergonovine (Ergotrate) is a generally well tolerated ergotamine derivative. Ergonovine is occasionally helpful for both cluster and migraine headache. The usual dose is 0.2 mg two to four times a day. Ergotrate is available as a 0.2 mg pill, but limited quantities are stocked in most pharmacies. Compounding pharmacists can formulate capsules of ergonovine in any desired strength. Similar long term restrictions and cautions apply to ergonovine as apply to methysergide or other ergotamines. Side effects, such as nausea and anxiety, are similar to those of the other ergotamines. Ergonovine may be helpful because it often is better tolerated than methysergide or standard ergotamines.

Steroid Blockade of the Occipital Nerve

By placing cortisone in the region of the greater occipital nerve, we often provide days to weeks of decreased cluster headache. This therapy is utilized at the peak of the cluster series if the headaches are poorly controlled. An injection may be repeated once, if necessary, but two injections per cluster series is the absolute maximum that I will utilize. I do not use more than two occipital cortisone injections per year in a patient.

I usually use 60 to 80 mg of Depo-Medrol per injection. Betamethasone may be used, but the Depo-Medrol may provide longer relief from the clusters. A thin needle (25 gauge) is preferred. For the technique of occipital nerve injection, please see Chapter 13.

Third Line Preventive Medication for Episodic Clusters

Third line strategies include: IV DHE, administered repetitively, and intranasal cocaine solution, used during the day to prevent the clusters.

Intravenous DHE

Intravenous DHE is useful for quickly decreasing the number of cluster headaches. It is necessary to follow the DHE with preventive medication, such as verapamil or lithium. I give the DHE in the office in a series of three to six injections of 1 mg each. This may be done in the hospital, but the office procedure is much more convenient for the patient.

IV DHE often allows us to control the clusters while waiting for the preventive medication to take effect. At times it is effective for weeks, or until the end of the cluster cycle. At times it is effective for weeks, or until the end of the cluster cycle. This procedure may be repeated during one cluster period. If the patient has received three to six injections of DHE intravenously, they may receive more DHE later in the cycle, if necessary. The intravenous protocol is completely discussed in Chapter 3.

Intranasal Cocaine Solution to Prevent Cluster Headaches

If the episodic cluster series is several months long, and all other preventive measures have not been effective, cocaine is an alternative. The prophylactic administration of a 10% solution during the day often reduces the number and severity of the clusters. Cocaine is useful for chronic cluster sufferers, particularly during the "peak" season of their headaches. Patients need to be screened carefully for any potential for addiction. If they have experienced any problem with addictive drugs, I do not use this treatment. This is a last resort.

The 10% solution of cocaine rarely produces euphoric or cognitive effects, and the total amount of cocaine that the patient uses in 1 or 2 months is small, from 1 to 2 g. Cocaine is often effective when other measures have not helped. However, with the addiction potential, the cost of the drops, and the difficulty in obtaining the solution, I consider this to be a "last resort", end of the line therapy.

The usual dose of the cocaine is one or two drops in each nostril one to four times a day. If the clusters are severe and out of control, I will begin with two drops four times a day, and we quickly decrease the dose down to as little as is effective. I usually give a triplicate script for a 10% cocaine solution, 10 or 20 cc. This is not refillable. If the patient shows any sign of overuse, I will not write another script. The cocaine is usually limited to 20 cc in a 2 month period, which is 2 g of cocaine in 2 months. Patients can occasionally achieve the same effect from a 4% solution of cocaine, but it is easier to simply titrate the amount of 10% drops down to one per day.

Side effects of the cocaine are not usually encountered with this strength. Patients may feel nervous, or insomnia can become a problem. The euphoric effects of cocaine may occur, but these are not common. If patients do experience euphoria, we need to decrease the percentage of the cocaine to 4%, or stop the treatment completely. The idea behind this end of the line treatment is to decrease the clusters, not to produce cocaine-addicted patients.

Miscellaneous Therapies for Prevention of Episodic Cluster Headache

In the occasional patient, various other medications are helpful for their cluster headaches. These include indomethacin, phenelzine, cyproheptadine, nifedipine, and beta blockers such as propranolol.

Indomethacin (Indocin) is discussed in Chapter 13. It is an anti-inflammatory that occasionally will decrease cluster headaches, but indomethacin is much more helpful in the cluster variant, chronic paroxysmal hemicrania (Chapter 13). The usual dose ranges from 75 to 225 mg per day.

Phenelzine (Nardil) is an MAO inhibitor that is a powerful antimigraine medication. Phenelzine is discussed in Chapter 3. Cluster patients occasionally respond to phenelzine, but this medication is more useful in severe migraine and daily headache patients when the standard treatments are ineffective.

Cyproheptadine (Periactin) is occasionally helpful for clusters, but the effect is usually very mild. The side effects of fatigue and weight gain often are a problem. Cyproheptadine is best used as adjunctive therapy for clusters that are poorly controlled.

Nifedipine (Procardia) is a well tolerated calcium blocker that is as effective as verapamil for many cluster patients. However, if verapamil does not work, the nifedipine usually is ineffective. The usual dose is 60 mg per day, and Procardia is available in capsules of 10 or 20 mg, and sustained release 30 mg (Procardia XL). Procardia is usually dosed two to three times per day. Side effects are very similar to verapamil.

Beta blockers are, at times, effective for cluster patients. They are much less effective, in general, than the usual cluster therapies. Propranolol (Inderal) or nadolol (Corgard) may be used. These are discussed at length in Chapter 3.

Preventive Medication for Chronic Cluster Headache

The preventive medication approach for chronic cluster headache closely follows that for episodic clusters. All of the following medications have been discussed in the preceeding sections on preventive therapy for episodic cluster headache. For patients who have severe clusters that are refractive to conventional therapy, surgical techniques, either radiofrequency trigeminal rhizotomy or glycerol injections (Retrogasserian), are options to be considered.

First line chronic cluster preventives include verapamil, lithium, and valproate (Depakote). If one of these three is not effective, we then use polypharmacy, by combining two or, occasionally, all three of the first line medications together.

There are many second line medications for chronic clusters. These include cortisone, daily ergotamines, methysergide (Sansert), ergonovine, and steroid blockade of the occipital nerve. Cortisone is used primarily during the "peak" time for the clusters, and cortisone is usually limited to 1 or 2 weeks duration. Daily ergots are occasionally effective, and the rebound headache situation rarely occurs with clusters. Sansert or ergonovine are more helpful and effective for episodic clusters, but certain chronic cluster patients do respond to these medications. Steroid block-ade around the greater occipital nerve, ipsilateral to the cluster pain, may provide weeks or, occasionally, months of relief. However, this technique is more useful for episodic clusters. All of these medications are discussed above in the episodic cluster prevention sections.

Third line medications for chronic clusters are the same as for episodic clusters. Intravenous DHE and cocaine nasal drops are the third line therapies, and these are discussed above in the episodic cluster section. Because of the inconvenience and cost of these treatments, and the addiction potential of the cocaine, these approaches are usually used only for very refractive patients.

Miscellaneous treatments for chronic clusters are the same as for episodic clusters: indomethacin (Indocin), phenelzine (Nardil), cypro-heptadine (Periactin), nifedipine (Procardia), and beta blockers (pro-pranolol, nadolol). These are occasionally helpful, and are discussed in the preceeding section on preventive medications for episodic clusters.

Surgical treatment for chronic clusters is a viable option if the patient has been refractive to medical management. The patient usually needs to suffer strictly unilateral pain. The primary technique that has been employed is radiofrequency trigeminal rhizotomy. The major risk is cor-neal anesthesia. The procedure may fail, or the surgery may need to be repeated. However, the results have been impressive. This radiofrequency procedure has been accomplished primarily in Houston, Texas, under the supervision of Dr. Ninan Mathew.

An alternative surgical procedure is retrogasserian injections of glyc-erol. In the limited number of patients who have undergone this treatment at the Cleveland Clinic, corneal safety has been achieved. The results have been promising with this technique, but only small numbers of patients have had the glycerol injected.

CHAPTER 11

Cluster Headache
Sample Case Studies

Case #1: 40-Year-Old Man with Episodic Clusters

Richard is a 40-year-old man with a history of 4 weeks of cluster headache once each year. These began when he was 35 years old. His cluster periods occur in the fall. The cluster period begins slowly, increasing over 1 week, reaching a peak where Richard has two or three severe cluster attacks each day. They occur from 10 p.m. to 3 a.m. Each cluster headache lasts from 40 to 90 minutes, and the headaches are severe. The pain is always on the right side, with eye tearing and nasal congestion.

Richard comes into our office 1 week into this fall's cluster series. The headaches are increasing in intensity, and he is miserable with the pain. At this point, we want to place Richard on a prophylactic regimen, and give him an abortive that may ease the acute attack. We decide to use 20 mg tablets of prednisone, one in the morning and one with dinner, or 40 mg per day for 4 days. We will reduce this to 20 mg per day in 4 days, and then to 10 mg per day in another 6 days. We will then taper off prednisone over another 4 to 6 days. Limiting the amount of corticosteroids is important for two reasons: (1) serious side effects are decreased, and (2) if necessary, we may utilize additional cortisone later in the cluster period. If the patient has been on high dose steroids for 3 weeks, we cannot use more cortisone. However, if we have kept the amount to a minimum, we are able to utilize the steroids later in the cluster period.

At the same time as the cortisone, we begin verapamil in the slow release form (Isoptin SR 240 mg, or Calan SR 240 mg). This is started at one per day, and with Richard we may eventually go up to two per day, which is generally the maximum (480 mg per day). Hopefully, by the time the prednisone is being decreased and weaned off, the verapamil will be effective.

As an abortive, we discuss the use of oxygen with Richard. He wants to wait on this. We give him Ergostat SL tablets, as he is reluctant to begin self-injecting DHE or sumatriptan. Richard has no risk factors for ergots. He will take one Ergostat, sublingually or swallowed, at the onset of the cluster. Richard is also instructed to apply ice to the area of pain.

Six days later, Richard calls; he had 5 very good days, but as the prednisone is being decreased, the headaches are becoming more severe. Ergostat does not help, and last night he had 90 minutes of extreme, intense pain. At this point we convince Richard to try oxygen, 8 liters per minute, as needed, and he rents a tank. I also obtain for Richard one plastic spray bottle filled with 4% topical lidocaine, to use as needed on the side of the pain. He is to lie supine, turn his head toward the side of the pain, and extend his head backwards. He will then spray two or three sprays of the lidocaine intranasally, as needed for the pain. Although lidocaine is only minimally effective for cluster headache, side effects are minimal. If it gives 25% relief the lidocaine is worthwhile. Richard is given sumatriptan (Imitrex) and taught how to utilize the injections.

I continue the original plan of decreasing prednisone, and I increase the verapamil to 480 mg per day (2 of the SR 240 mg tablets per day). We will check Richard's blood pressure. The Ergostat did not help, and he now has oxygen, Imitrex, and lidocaine. Lithium or Sansert are considerations. IV DHE (4 injections in the office) or a cortisone injection around the occipital nerve are possibilities. The injection would be on the side of the pain. In addition, daily ergotamine, 2 mg each night, may be effective.

I see Richard 4 days later. He is now in his third week of clusters, and based on his previous cluster episodes, he has 1 or 2 more weeks left in this cycle. However, at times the cluster period may exceed the previous one, and extended cluster periods may occur, sometimes lasting months. Richard states that oxygen helps, but lidocaine does not. The clusters are less severe but continue at two per night. Imitrex injections stop the clusters within 15 minutes. The verapamil may be having some effect. He is down to 20 mg per day of prednisone, and we decide to taper off the prednisone over the next 4 days. If the headaches increase dramatically, we could use more prednisone. Richard agrees to come into the office 2 days in a row for IV DHE, and I give him 4 mg total over the 2 days. He is in our office for only 3 hours each day. The DHE stops the clusters for 4 days, and then they return, but not nearly as severe. Six days later, the headaches are gone, and after 1 week without headaches, Richard is tapered off the verapamil over 6 days. If the headaches were to return during those 6 days, I would immediately increase the verapamil again, to 480 mg per day, and consider the use of prednisone.

It is important to chart which medications were effective for a patient's clusters, so as to be ready to use them for the next cluster series. I usually write in the chart the plan for the next series, and I inform the patient. In Richard's case, we would utilize oxygen as an abortive along with injections of sumatriptan. As preventive medication, we would use verapamil, increasing up to 480 mg per day, and he will be given approximately 2 weeks of prednisone. IV DHE may be worthwhile to use again with Richard, as this time it decreased the severity of the clusters during his "peak" period of headache.

Case #2: 58-Year-Old Woman with Episodic Clusters

Shelly is a 58-year-old woman with one or two cluster series per year, each lasting 6 to 13 weeks. Shelly began experiencing cluster headaches at age 34. She suffers two to three severe headaches per day, primarily early morning. Shelly has left sided clusters, with eye tearing and rhinorrhea, and significant nausea during the attack. The length of her attacks averages 45 minutes.

Shelly comes to our office 1 week into this cluster series. In the past, she has been refractive to indomethacin, cortisone, methysergide, and verapamil. Oxygen does help, but is only partially effective. This series is beginning to increase in intensity, and we need to institute effective preventive medication. The options are: lithium, valproate (Depakote), occipital nerve (steroid) injections, sumatriptan or DHE injections at home, or reinstituting verapamil along with another preventive.

For prophylactic therapy, we begin with lithium, 300 mg each night with dinner. The average dose of lithium for cluster patients is approximately 600 mg, which is a low dose. I will progress to 900 or 1,200 mg per day, at most. As an abortive, Shelly uses oxygen, and I give her a small bottle of 4% topical lidocaine. She does not wish to utilize an injection.

Three days later, Shelly calls stating that she is very nauseated and is experiencing mood swings with the lithium. I stop the lithium, as she is on only one per day, and could not tolerate more than this amount. We will need to switch preventives. She comes in for an occipital steroid injection. I give her 60 mg of Depo-Medrol on the ipsilateral (left) side. We begin Depakote, 250 mg twice per day, increasing in 3 days to 500 mg twice per day. Shelly states that the clusters are severe, and oxygen decreases the pain approximately 30%, but lidocaine does not help. We stop the lidocaine. As an abortive, DHE is a possibility, but Shelly does not wish to use an injection. The DHE nasal spray is occasionally helpful, but with cluster patients the nasal congestion tends to be exacerbated with DHE nasal spray. Ergotamine preparations, such as Ergostat or Cafergot, are usually not instituted in a person 58 years of age because of the cardiac risks. As an abortive, with the oxygen, I give Shelly Fiorinal, to take one or two at the onset of the cluster. Although pain medications are not ideal for clusters, at times they may be used, and they do give the patient some sense of control over the very intense pain. Narcotics or sedatives should be limited per week and per month.

One week later, Shelly comes into our office. She had 4 headache-free days after the occipital injection, and the headaches have been significantly milder for the past week. Shelly feels that Fiorinal did help to a small degree, but she became slightly nervous, presumably due to the caffeine. The Depakote makes her slightly tired. I stop the Fiorinal and substitute Axotal, which is the same as Fiorinal, without the caffeine. Axotal contains butalbital plus aspirin. Phrenilin, which is acetaminophen and butalbital, without caffeine, is a possibility. With these butalbital medications, it is important to use the brand name, not the generic, as the generic simply is not as effective.

Because of the Depakote, a c.b.c and SMA are drawn. I also check the valproate level, but at 1,000 mg per day the level will usually be low. Unlike the situation with epilepsy, we do not titrate the dose of Depakote to the blood level. Low doses of Depakote are often effective for headache.

Shelly's blood tests are normal, and she calls 10 days later. The headaches have been increasing, and she has one severe cluster each night. The Depakote remains partially effective, because Shelly usually has two severe clusters per night. The Axotal and oxygen provide partial relief. At this juncture, I increase the Depakote from 1,000 to 1,500 mg per day. Shelly takes 500 mg in the morning and 1,000 mg with dinner.

Five days later, Shelly reports that the clusters are mild, but she is very lethargic and nauseated on the 1,500 mg of Depakote. I drop the Depakote back to 500 mg twice per day (1,000 mg per day total). We recheck the SMA (blood test), and the liver functions are normal. I add verapamil once again. Although verapamil had previously failed to decrease Shelly's headaches, it may be effective in combination with the Depakote. We are now utilizing verapamil plus Depakote as prophylactic therapy. I begin with verapamil SR (either Calan SR, 240 mg, or Isoptin SR, 240 mg), once per day.

One week later, Shelly reports that the side effects from the Depakote are gone on the lower dose of 1,000 mg. She tolerates the verapamil well. However, Shelly is beginning to experience one very severe cluster each night, and she states that she cannot tolerate the pain. The Axotal does not help. Cluster patients often become desperate due to the excruciating pain. We teach Shelly to self-inject with sumatriptan.

Four days later, Shelly reports that the sumatriptan was effective. This decreased the pain approximately 50%, and with the oxygen, she was able to control the pain. Shelly was very nauseated with the injection. I give her Tigan, 250 mg PO, to take with the sumatriptan. She does not wish to use a suppository. Shelly remains on the Depakote and verapamil.

Over the next 10 days, the clusters wind down and decrease in severity. Shelly has one mild to moderate headache per day. I recheck the blood tests because of the verapamil and Depakote.

One week later, the clusters are gone. We stop verapamil and Depakote over 1 week. Shelly is instructed that if the clusters return, she should restart the verapamil at one per day. The Depakote would also be started again. For the next series we will use the following medications, as they have been somewhat useful for this series: (1) Depakote, 1,000 mg per day, (2) Calan or Isoptin SR, 240 mg, one per day, (3) occipital nerve injections, (4) Oxygen PRN, and (5) sumatriptan injections with Tigan for nausea. Shelly could not tolerate lithium. If the headaches are refractive in the future, alternative possibilities include: IV DHE (at least 4 injections), increasing verapamil to 480 mg per day, daily ergotamines or ergonovine, and intranasal cocaine, used during the cluster cycle as a preventive medication. Cocaine would be a "last resort" approach, but it is usually effective.

Case #3: 34-Year-Old Man with Severe Chronic Cluster Headache

Michael is a 34-year-old man with a history since age 25 of one or two right sided cluster headaches per day. He experiences occasional breaks of one or two months without headache. The clusters vary in severity, and usually last 1 hour. They are increased in spring and fall. Michael's headaches occur at any time of the day or night, but tend to occur more between the hours of 9 and 11 p.m. He has no other medical problems.

Michael has been refractive to propranolol, sinus medications, and verapamil. Oxygen helps approximately 50%. Lidocaine does not help. Steroids have provided temporary benefit. Sumatriptan gave Michael chest discomfort, and he does not wish to use sumatriptan again.

We decide to place Michael on lithium as a preventive. Alternative considerations for preventive medication include valproate (Depakote), methysergide (Sansert), daily ergotamine, IV DHE, indomethacin, and intranasal cocaine drops. Surgery, such as radiofrequency rhizotomy, is becoming a more viable option for chronic cluster patients refractive to medication. We begin with one 300 mg lithium carbonate pill with dinner, and after several days increase this to one pill twice per day. As an abortive, oxygen is continued, and we give Michael Ergostat SL tablets, to use under the tongue as needed. He may simply swallow the Ergostat, as this is usually as effective as the sublingual route.

Michael comes into the office several weeks later for a blood test. The headaches are improved on the lithium but the Ergostat makes him nauseated, and he states it did not sufficiently abort the headache. We may eventually utilize Ergostat to prevent the headaches. Michael has had only two headaches in the past week.

With chronic cluster headaches, the patients usually have certain seasons of headache exacerbation. Michael experiences increased cluster headaches in August, and we are now in the beginning of August. The headaches are increasing, and we increase the lithium to three per day.

This is usually as much as I will use with lithium, but I will occasionally push it to 1,200 mg per day (4 of the 300 mg pills). As an abortive, Michael learns to give himself IM injections of DHE. He is to limit these to a maximum of four per week.

Two weeks later, we check the routine blood tests, along with a lithium level, and everything is normal. The headaches have diminished to one per day, and the DHE is somewhat effective. Michael continues to experience limited relief from oxygen. However, he is very tremulous on the lithium, and does not feel that he can tolerate three per day. We reduce the lithium to two per day.

On two lithium, the headaches are increased once again to two per day. The oxygen and DHE help, but he still has 30 minutes of severe pain each night. The anticipation of the severe nightly headache is very depressing to cluster patients. As we cannot increase the lithium, we now switch to Depakote, and the lithium is discontinued. Depakote is generally more effective for chronic cluster than methysergide (Sansert), and there is less concern over long term side effects. Methysergide is occasionally effective for episodic clusters. I give Michael 250 mg tablets of Depakote, to take twice per day with food for the first 4 days. He will then increase to 500 mg twice per day. We decide to utilize the outpatient IV DHE protocol.

I give Michael four injections of IV DHE over 2 days. Each injection is 1 mg, and we administer the DHE in our office, not in the hospital. The headaches improve with the DHE, and he continues on the Depakote. Depakote may take 3 or 4 weeks to become effective, and we may need to increase the dose. He is slightly fatigued with the Depakote, and Michael experiences mild gastritis. We add Pepcid, 20 mg, to take daily with the Depakote. Generally I do not like to add more medication to counter side effects, but with Michael our options are limited. We need to give the Depakote time to become effective.

The headaches were improved for 2 weeks after the IV DHE, but they are now increasing. We are in September, which is usually a bad month for Michael's headaches. I check the blood tests, and they are normal. Michael is on 1,000 mg per day of Depakote, and his GI symptoms are alleviated on Pepcid. I attempt to push the Depakote to 1,500 mg per day, one 500 mg tablet in the morning, and two tablets with dinner. He is nauseated after the dinner dose, and we then change the schedule to one 500 mg pill three times a day.

If Michael was not experiencing GI upset, we could utilize small amounts of cortisone. Although cortisone is usually reserved for episodic clusters, small amounts often aid the chronic cluster patient during difficult periods.

Michael states that the headaches are improved with the 1,500 mg of Depakote, but he continues to experience one severe cluster at approximately 10 p.m. each night. The headache lasts 45 minutes. I give him

Ergostat to take sublingually each night at 9 p.m. At times, ergotamine taken prior to the expected onset of the cluster will prevent the cluster headache. The rebound headache situation due to ergotamines is not usually a problem with cluster patients, and we can use daily ergotamine. Since Michael has been utilizing IM DHE, I ask him to discontinue the DHE while on Ergostat.

The Ergostat does help but he is very nauseated with it. Michael does not wish to continue ergotamine on a daily basis. Michael does not feel he can handle more Depakote, as he has gastritis on the 1,500 mg per day. After discontinuing the Ergostat, for prevention Michael is only on the Depakote. He uses oxygen and DHE abortively.

Michael continues this regimen through the winter, with one headache per night that is partially controlled with oxygen, and occasionally he utilizes the DHE injections. In April his headaches increase dramatically, and Michael suffers through two very severe ones per day. The Depakote is no longer effective. We discuss the possibility of a surgical procedure, radiofrequency rhizotomy, that has had moderate success with chronic cluster patients. He is not eager to pursue this, and wishes to proceed with medication. At this point, the Depakote is discontinued, but it is possible that Depakote may be effective again in the future. Since the headaches are very severe, I administer four more injections of IV DHE in our office.

In addition to the IV DHE, I give Michael an occipital nerve injection of Depo-Medrol, 60 mg. This is done on the right side, ipsilateral to Michael's pain. He has been refractive to lithium, daily ergotamine, verapamil, and Depakote. These may work in combination with one another, but at present we have two options: (1) methysergide (Sansert), and (2) intranasal cocaine, used daily to prevent the clusters. Methysergide is only mildly effective for most chronic cluster patients; cocaine is much more effective. However, cocaine has only limited utility because of the cost, the difficulty in obtaining the solution, and its addiction potential.

The IV DHE and occipital injection help Michael for 2 weeks; the clusters are less severe and last only 20 minutes. We place Michael on methysergide (Sansert), 2 mg, one pill with food each day. He feels hot and flushed, and experiences a mild increase in gastritis. Michael takes Pepcid once again for the gastritis. With methysergide, side effects such as nausea and facial flushing usually diminish if the patient is able to continue the medication.

With the methysergide, the DHE is discontinued. The one pill per day decreases the headaches by 25%, and we attempt to increase the dose to two per day. Michael experiences severe GI pain, with dizziness and nausea. Methysergide is now decreased back to one per day. It is now June, which is typically one of the better months for Michael's clusters.

In August the headaches increase, and the methysergide is no longer effective. Michael receives four additional injections of IV DHE, providing 1 week of relief. A repeat occipital steroid injection is a consideration, but these should be given in limited numbers. I stop the methysergide, and place Michael on cocaine drops. He has never had a problem with addicting drugs or alcohol, and Michael understands the problems with cocaine. Patients need to be carefully screened for addiction potential prior to utilizing cocaine. It is truly an "end of the line, last resort" approach. Michael is desperate with the clusters, experiencing two severe headaches per day. The total amount of cocaine that the patients receive is actually small, approximately 1 g or less per month. With the 10% cocaine solution that is utilized, most patients do not experience euphoria, insomnia, or anxiety. Patients may be weaned down to a 4% solution, but this is usually ineffective. I give Michael 10 cc of a 10% solution of cocaine, as a triplicate script. He is to take one drop in each nostril three to four times per day; we adjust this up or down, depending on the response. Some patients require one or two drops per day, and others require two drops four times a day, in each nostril. Patients usually decrease the dose to the minimum amount necessary to aid the clusters. We periodically stop the cocaine, and only use it during a severe "peak" cluster season. If a patient exhibits any sign of overuse, the drops are discontinued.

Michael finds that the cocaine helps, and he uses one drop in each nostril three times per day. He has mild insomnia from this, but no other effects. We discuss the problems with cocaine, and decide to utilize it only during his peak cluster periods. After 3 months, we stop the cocaine, and restart Depakote, 500 mg three times a day. Possibilities in the future with Michael include additional cocaine drops, IV DHE, repeat occipital injections, and surgery. He continues to find the oxygen and IM DHE helpful as cluster abortives.

CHAPTER 12

Headache in Children and Adolescents

The following gives a practical guideline to headache therapy in children and adolescents. Many drugs that are helpful for headache have not recieved a specific FDA indication for this use, and often these have not been specifically approved for children. The risks, side effects, and problems associated with medications need to be fully explained to the family, as explained in the PDR or a similar reference. Only if the family understands the risks and side effects of a medication, and accepts these potential problems, is a medication given to the child. See Chapter 1 for a general discussion of migraine.

Introduction

Headache is a common complaint among children and adolescents. The generally stated incidence of migraine at age 6 is 1%, and at age 10 is 4%. These figures may be low. Migraine is a problem in children as young as ages 2 or 3. Gathering accurate data in this age group is exceedingly difficult, as parents usually attribute headaches and nausea to "the flu". Migraine in children and adolescents, and chronic daily headache (CDH) in adolescents, is a major problem, with much lost school time caused by migraine or daily headache. Depression is common in adolescents with severe, frequent headaches, and in many cases the depression is caused by the headaches. Approaching headaches in children and adolescents with counseling, biofeedback-relaxation, and group therapy may be beneficial.

As with adults, the vast majority of the time we are dealing with either migraine or tension headache (if this is daily, we would term it chronic daily headache, or CDH). Organic etiologies need to be excluded, of course, and an MRI scan of the brain is necessary once in the life of most of the younger patients with frequent, severe headaches. Organic pathology, the pediatric neurologic history, and the pediatric neurologic physical exam are beyond the scope of this book. I assume in this book that the diagnosis of tension headache or migraine has been firmly estab-

TABLE 12.1. Migraine in Childhood: Clinical Features.

Lack of sleep is a major trigger factor in children with
  migraine
Insomnia occurs more often in children with headache
Migraine often decreases or stops by age 20, particularly in
  males
Vomiting occurs early in the headache
Male prevalence is slightly greater than female, which is the
  opposite in adults
Headaches do not last as long as in adults
Head trauma may precipitate migraine
Increased incidence of epilepsy

lished. Basilar artery migraine occurs more frequently in the adolescent age range than in adults. The symptoms are brain stem, cerebellar, and occipital lobe in origin, and the headache is more likely to be in the occiput. Dizziness, slurred speech, paralysis, ataxia, vertigo, brief loss of consciousness, partial visual field loss, blurry vision, stupor, nausea, and vomiting may all occur. (See Table 12.1).

All of the usual migraine trigger factors, such as diet, should be discussed with the patient and family. These are extensively discussed in Chapter 1. Relaxation/biofeedback should be given to younger patients with frequent headache. Most children cannot learn and apply biofeedback before the age of 9, but some 7 or 8 year olds can learn simple breathing and imaging techniques that may help their headaches. Peer groups or individual counseling for the adolescent and parents are often helpful. The incidence of hard driving, perfectionistic behavior, and depression is increased in adolescents with severe headache. Children and adolescents may be in too many activities and feel extremely stressed. These issues need to be addressed. Children missing substantial blocks of time in school need to be assessed for depression or school phobia.

We have two types of medication therapy: abortive and preventive. The decision as to how much medication to use depends upon the frequency and severity of the headaches and how much they bother the child. Some children are simply not bothered by their daily headaches and tend to simply ignore them. Others may be incapacitated and miss an entire year of school. As with adult headache patients, in children and adolescents, abortive medication is used in the overwhelming majority of cases, without daily preventive medication. However, with frequent migraines that are more than mild, or moderate to severe daily headaches, daily preventive medication may be necessary. It is always reasonable to try biofeedback as the first step, with simple abortive medications, and attempt to avoid daily preventive medication.

When I do use preventive medication with children and adolescents, I always attempt to stop the preventive medication periodically, and to minimize medication. As with adults, the idea is to see if we may return to simply using abortive medication.

Abortive Medication for Children Less Than 11 Years Old

Tension Headache

We generally do not "chase" after tension headaches all day with pain-killers; limited amounts of acetaminophen or ibuprofen are acceptable. However, if the child has headaches on a daily basis that are severe enough to require more than a minimal amount of painkiller, the preventive medication needs to be considered. For sporadic tension headaches, or mild to moderate daily headaches, we do use limited amounts of acetaminophen, ibuprofen, or caffeine. As with most types of headache, a dark, quiet room and ice to the head is usually beneficial.

Acetaminophen

This well tolerated medication is safe in children but not as effective as ibuprofen or aspirin. The dose is usually 5 to 10 mg/kg per dose, with a maximum per day of 30 or 40 mg/kg. Alternatively, the dose at age 4 to 5 is 240 mg each time, at age 6 to 8 it is 320 mg, at age 9 to 10 it is 400 mg, and at age 11 it is 480 mg. Five doses per 24 hours should be the maximum. Acetaminophen may be given every 2 to 4 hours. Acetaminophen will rarely produce side effects, but fatigue is occasionally seen. Chewable, liquid, and suppository forms are available. These render acetaminophen very versatile for this age group. If children require more than one dose per day of acetaminophen, then preventive medication needs to be considered. Adding a small amount of caffeine, in the form of a caffeinated soft drink, may enhance the effectiveness of the acetaminophen. Aspirin free Excedrin combines acetaminophen with 65 mg of

---

TABLE 12.2. Quick Reference Guide: Abortive Medications for Tension Headache in Children.

1. Acetaminophen: Well tolerated, safe, not as effective as ibuprofen or aspirin. Chewable tablets and liquid are available. The usual dose is 5 to 10 mg/kg per dose. Because of safety, acetaminophen is the usual primary abortive medication to utilize in children. The addition of caffeine may enhance the effectiveness.
2. Ibuprofen: More effective than acetaminophen, but with occasional GI upset. Liquid Advil is available, which helps in younger children. Caffeine may enhance the effectiveness. The usual dose is 100 to 200 mg. Effective for migraine as well as tension headache.
3. Caffeine: Either used by itself, or with an analgesic, caffeine is useful for tension and migraine headache. In children, soft drinks containing caffeine are helpful. Side effects are minimal when caffeine is used in very limited amounts.

caffeine; this is more useful for migraine than for daily headache. Forms of acetaminophen available are: Chewable tablets, 80, 120, and 160 mg. Regular (non-chewable) tablets, 325, 500, and 650 mg. Capsules, 325 and 500 mg. Syrup, 80, 120, 160, and 325 mg per 5 cc (teaspoon). There is also a Tylenol Extra Strength liquid with 500 mg per 15 ml (3 teaspoons). Suppositories are available in strengths of 120, 125, 325, 600, and 650 mg. Finally, there is a bromo seltzer product with buffered acetaminophen that contains 325 mg of acetaminophen (per $\frac{3}{4}$ capful measure), sodium bicarbonate, and citric acid.

Ibuprofen

Ibuprofen is harsher on the GI tract, liver, and kidneys than is acetaminophen, but is generally more effective. Side effects include GI upset or pain, nausea, fatigue, and occasionally dizziness. Ibuprofen is, however, well tolerated in the vast majority of children. Allergic or anaphylactic reactions may occur but are not common. If used daily, renal and hepatic function needs to be monitored periodically. Adding a small amount of caffeine to the ibuprofen, in the form of a caffeinated soft drink, may enhance efficacy.

The dose for abortive use is as follows: Age 4 to 5; 100 mg (1 teaspoon of the children's Advil liquid, which is 100 mg per 5 ml) every 3 to 4 hours as needed. Do not exceed 40 mg per kg per day. Age 6 to 8; 100 to 150 mg (1 to $1\frac{1}{2}$ teaspoons) every 3 to 4 hours as needed. Do not exceed 40 mg per kg per day. Age 9 to 10; 150 to 200 mg per dose. The 200 mg tablets may be used if the child is able to swallow tablets. Do not exceed 40 mg per kg per day. Age 11 to 12; 200 to 400 mg per dose, do not exceed 40 mg per kg per day. Ibuprofen is available in the following forms: Tablets, 200 mg (or, by prescription, 400 mg). Liquid: Children's Advil, 100 mg per 5 cc.

Caffeine

Caffeine is effective for many patient's headaches, and it appears in many headache medications (Anacin, Excedrin, Vanquish). Small amounts of caffeine are helpful for children's headaches; one-half or a whole caffeinated soft drink will enhance the effectiveness of many headache abortives, or the caffeine may be effective simply used by itself.

Migraine Headache

A dark room, sleep, and ice to the head often help alleviate the pain of a migraine headache. When nausea is a prominent feature in the child, we either must simply wait for the nausea to abate, or for the child to vomit, and then use an abortive, or we can utilize an antiemetic. Rectal suppositories are more effective than oral medication in migraineurs, and

---

TABLE 12.3. Quick Reference Guide: First Line Migraine Abortives in Children.

1. Ibuprofen, Acetaminophen, Caffeine: Ibuprofen is effective and available as a liquid, but GI upset is relatively common. Acetaminophen is very safe, less effective than the other abortives, but easy to use, with liquid and chewable forms available. For children who are nauseated and cannot swallow oral medication, compounding pharmacists are able to formulate acetaminophen into a lozenge, to be kept in the mouth and absorbed by the buccal mucosa. This may be combined, in a lozenge, with an antiemetic such as Phenergan or Tigan. Caffeine decreases migraine pain in most children, and may be used alone, or in combination with other abortives.
2. Naproxen (Naprosyn, Anaprox): Naproxen is an effective abortive that is nonsedating and is available as a liquid. GI side effects are very common, however. Adding small amounts of caffeine, such as in soft drinks, may enhance the effectiveness.
3. Midrin: These are very large capsules that consist of a combination of a nonaddicting sedative, acetaminophen, and a vasoconstrictor. The capsules may be taken apart, and the Midrin swallowed with applesauce or juice. Sedation is common, as is lightheadedness. GI upset, although not very frequent, occurs at times.

---

with severe nausea, oral medications are not well tolerated. Oral lozenges of Tigan or Phenergan may be formulated by compounding pharmacists. Many parents are reluctant to use suppositories with their child, and thus it is often best to wait for the nausea to subside, or use oral lozenges. Compounding pharmacists can put together oral lozenges for children, in any flavor, with almost any analgesic or antiemetic medication. If nausea is not prominent, the migraine is much easier to treat with medication. The earlier the medication is given, the more effective it tends to be.

The first line migraine abortives in children 10 years and under include caffeine, acetaminophen, ibuprofen, naproxen (Naprosyn, Anaprox), and Midrin. Butalbital compounds and aspirin comprise the second line therapy. Third line therapy, used in very unusual circumstances, are the corticosteroids and DHE-45 injections, either IV or IM. I have not found the standard ergots, other than DHE, to be useful in more than a few patients in this age group, primarily because of side effects. In addition, I have generally found the narcotics, such as codeine, to be helpful in only a very small minority of pediatric patients. Most children seem to feel ill with these, and we tend to exacerbate the situation with the use of narcotics.

First Line Migraine Abortives

Caffeine, Acetaminophen, and Ibuprofen

The mainstay of migraine therapy for children under age 11 remains acetaminophen, because of its safety and lack of side effects. However, it is less effective than the other migraine abortives. Combining acetaminophen with caffeine may enhance efficacy (for instance, taking Tylenol with Coke or Pepsi). Aspirin Free Excedrin combines the acetaminophen with 65 mg of caffeine; this is helpful for those 9 or 10 year olds who can tolerate this dose of caffeine. Ibuprofen is more effective, but also much more likely to produce gastric irritation. Ibuprofen should be taken with food. The fact that ibuprofen is available in liquid form eases dosing. Acetaminophen is also available OTC as a liquid; Advil by prescription only. The suppositories are, at times, helpful, but we are reluctant to use rectal suppositories with children. Oral lozenges of acetaminophen may be formulated by a compounding pharmacist, and these sit in the buccal mucosa to be absorbed. They can be flavored for the children. Tigan or Phenergan may be added to the lozenge for antiemetic purposes. For full information on caffeine, acetaminophen, and ibuprofen, see above section on tension abortives.

Naproxen (Naprosyn, Anaprox)

Naproxen is widely used as an abortive migraine medication in adults. Liquid Naprosyn is helpful, as many children will not swallow pills. GI side effects are common, and sedation occasionally occurs. If naproxen is used on a daily basis, renal and hepatic functions need to be monitored. Naproxen appears to somewhat more effective than acetaminophen or ibuprofen. Using naproxen with small amounts of caffeine may enhance the efficacy.

Naproxen is dosed in children according to weight: At 30 lb, we would start with $\frac{1}{2}$ teaspoon of the suspension (125 mg per 5 ml), or about 62 mg, and this may be repeated only once in the day. At 55 lb, we would use one teaspoon (5 cc), or 125 mg, and this may be repeated once only. At 85 lb, we use 1 to 1.5 teaspoons, or 125 to 185 mg per dose, and this may be repeated once only. Alternatively, one half of the Naprosyn 250 mg pill may be used. For children over 100 lb, the Anaprox 275 mg (which is equivalent in naproxen to a 250 mg pill of Naprosyn) may be used.

Oral Lozenges Formulated by Compounding Pharmacists

Medication such as acetaminophen may be formulated into a palatable lozenge, to be absorbed by the buccal mucosa. Many children cannot swallow oral medication, or they are very nauseated with migraines, and we generally do not want to utilize rectal suppositories in children. As antiemetics, Tigan or Phenergan may be used as an oral lozenge.

Midrin

Midrin capsules have 325 mg of acetaminophen, 65 mg of isometheptane mucate (a mild vasoconstrictor), and 100 mg of dichloralphenazone, a mild nonaddicting sedative. The generic Midrin does not work as well. Sedation and lightheadedness are common with Midrin, and GI upset is occasionally seen. Midrin is reasonably effective in migraine, and may be used as young as age 7. The capsules are large, and they may be pulled apart, with the ingredients put into applesauce. At age 7 and 8, I start with one fourth or one half of a capsule, repeated every 2 hours if necessary, limited to two full capsules per day at most. At age 9 and 10, I start with one-half or one capsule, repeated if necessary at 2 hour intervals, three per day at most. Midrin has been used at times as a suppository, with pinholes punched into the capsule, but I have not found this to be helpful. Midrin is usually a second choice after acetaminophen, NSAIDs, and caffeine.

Second Line Abortive Medication

The two second line abortive medications are butalbital compounds and aspirin. The ergots and narcotics do not seem to be helpful in this age group. The butalbital compounds are helpful because they help to control the migraine and at the same time provide sedation. They are usually well tolerated. Butalbital compounds are discussed extensively in Chapter 2.

Butalbital Compounds

Butalbital compounds are extremely effective medications and include Fiorinal, Esgic, Esgic Plus, Fioricet, Axotal, Phrenilin, and Phrenilin Forte. The generic compounds do not work as well as the brand names, which is true for most of the migraine abortives. In general, Fiorinal is more effective than Esgic, which is more effective than Phrenilin. Each of these different compounds has a role in abortive therapy.

Fiorinal

Fiorinal contains 50 mg of butalbital, 325 mg of aspirin, and 40 mg of caffeine. The tablets may be cut in half for pediatric use. The sedative effect of butalbital is usually offset by the caffeine. Fiorinal is more effective than Esgic, because aspirin is more effective than acetaminophen. With varicella or influenza, the aspirin needs to be avoided because of the danger of Reye's syndrome. Dosage at age 7 and 8 begins with one-half tablet that may be repeated every 1 to 2 hours, up to a maximum of one tablet per day at most. I do not generally exceed this dose in this age group. At age 9 and 10, I will begin with one-half or one tablet, and this may be repeated in 3 hours, with a maximum of two tablets per day at most. Fatigue is a common side effect, and occasionally, nervousness. Nausea or GI pain may occur because of the aspirin. Lightheadedness, dizziness, or euphoria may occur because of the butalbital.

Esgic, Fioricet

Esgic is the same as Fioricet; Esgic is available as capsules or pills, Fioricet only as pills. They contain 50 mg of butalbital, a short acting sedative, 325 mg of acetaminophen, and 40 mg of caffeine. Thus, they are the same as fiorinal, but with acetaminophen instead of aspirin. They are, therefore, less effective than Fiorinal, but better tolerated. The generic is best avoided. The Esgic or Fioricet tablets may be cut in half.

The dose is the same as for Fiorinal. Fatigue is a common side effect, and occasionally, nervousness. Nausea may occur, but is not as frequent as it is with Fiorinal. Lightheadedness, dizziness, and euphoria may occur. Esgic and Fioricet are, in general, very well tolerated.

Phrenilin

Phrenilin has the same composition as Esgic but without the caffeine. It contains 50 mg of butalbital and 325 mg of acetaminophen. Phrenilin is a pill that may be cut in half. Although less effective than Fiorinal or Esgic, Phrenilin is helpful for children who cannot take caffeine or aspirin. The dose is the same as for Fiorinal. Side effects are usually mild, with sedation being frequent. Lightheadedness, dizziness, and euphoria may occur.

Aspirin

Aspirin is a second line medication because of the fear of Reye's syndrome. If parents are warned not to give aspirin with varicella or influenza, in the presence of a fever, aspirin may be safely used. However, many parents are reluctant to use aspirin in any situation. GI upset is relatively common with aspirin, but otherwise aspirin is usually well tolerated. Combining aspirin with caffeine (Anacin, or simply adding a caffeinated soft drink to the aspirin) enhances effectiveness. Aspirin and ibuprofen are, in general, more effective than acetaminophen for headache. At age 6 to 8, the dose is 325 mg every 4 hours as needed. At age 9 and 10, the dose is 400 mg every 4 hours. Children's aspirin is available in 65, 75, and 81 mg tablets. Aspergum has 227.5 mg per tablet. In addition, tablets are available in the standard 325 mg dosage.

Third Line Abortive Therapy

In unusual circumstances, cortisone or DHE may be employed, in very limited doses for short periods of time. For severe, prolonged migraine, Prednisone (or Decadron) and DHE are the most effective measures, which is the same situation as in adults. Prednisone has the advantage of being available orally, whereas DHE needs to be given as an injection. Compounding pharmacists are helpful in treating children's migraine headaches, for they are able to formulate almost any abortive medication into a flavored lozenge for the child. Cortisone, analgesics, and anti-emetics may all be combined in a lozenge.

Prednisone

If the migraine has been prolonged and refractive, Prednisone may be given in an attempt to "break the cycle." Alternatively, small doses of Decadron may be utilized. The dose is small, usually 10 mg of Prednisone PO twice a day with food, as needed, for 1 or 2 days only. I usually limit it to 40 mg total for the migraine, and if the headache is improved with 10 or 20 mg, I instruct the parents to simply stop giving it. Side effects in these small doses are minimal, with anxiety or GI upset being relatively common. Fatigue, insomnia, and dizziness may occur. (See section on corticosteroids in Chapter 2.)

DHE

DHE is not well tolerated in this age group, but is usually effective, and, at times, is the only effective therapy. I have used it in ages 9 and up. The IV route is preferred, because IM administration is not easily tolerated by children, and the IV route is more effective and somewhat less painful. As with adults, an antiemetic usually needs to be given prior to the DHE, usually at least $\frac{1}{2}$ hour before the DHE. Trimethobenzamide (Tigan) or promethazine (Phenergan) are usually utilized to prevent the nausea. The trimethobenzamide (Tigan) is available as pediatric suppositories of 100 and 200 mg, and capsules of 100 and 250 mg. Dosage is usually 100 to 200 mg per dose. Promethazine is available in 12.5 and 25 mg tablets, as a 6.25 or 25 mg per 5 ml syrup, and as 12.5 and 25 mg suppositories. The usual dose is 12.5 to 25 mg per dose. Alternatively, the children's dose is 0.25 to 0.5 mg/kg per dose. If the child has such severe nausea that injections of antiemetics are necessary, then I avoid giving the DHE, as it will increase the severe nausea. Antiemetics can be formulated as a lozenge by compounding pharmacists.

The DHE is pushed as a one time dose of $\frac{1}{3}$ to $\frac{1}{2}$ mg intravenously. Nausea, lightheadedness, a feeling of heat about the head, muscle con-traction headache, and leg cramps may occur. I usually give only one dose in children, but for severe, refractory headache, two doses per day may be given. Avoiding a hep-lock, and simply using a venipuncture, will render the entire procedure less painful for the child. (DHE is also discussed in Chapters 2 and 3.)

Antiemetics

In children, I usually use either trimethobenzamide (Tigan), or prome-thazine (Phenergan). I attempt to avoid the use of prochlorperazine

(Compazine) because of its increased incidence of extrapyramidal side effects and anxiety. Compazine, however, is generally more effective than Tigan or Phenergan.

In many children with nausea and vomiting early in the migraine, it is best to simply let them vomit, and then give an abortive migraine medication. If they cannot keep an oral preparation down, we have little choice but to use a suppository. Many parents are reluctant to utilize suppositories. At times, an oral flavored antiemetic lozenge is helpful. These are formulated by compounding pharmacists. With prolonged nausea or vomiting, however, a suppository is usually necessary. This eases the nausea and provides needed sedation for the child. Sedation and sleep usually help migraines in all ages.

Trimethobenzamide (Tigan)

Tigan is given as 100 to 200 mg doses, every 4 hours, as needed. It is generally an extremely well tolerated antiemetic. Fatigue is relatively common. Hypotension, extrapyramidal reactions, blurred vision, disorientation, muscle cramps, and dizziness occur but are uncommon.

Tigan is available in capsules of 100 and 250 mg, suppositories of 100 and 200 mg, and in injectable form at 100 mg per ml. Tigan may be formulated as a flavored lozenge by a compounding pharmacist.

Promethazine (Phenergan)

This well tolerated medication causes sedation in many patients but has an extremely low incidence of extrapyramidal side effects. The sedation is helpful for inducing sleep. Hypotension, blurred vision, disorientation, and dizziness may occur but are not common. The usual adult dose is 12.5 to 25 mg per dose, which may be repeated if necessary. In children it may be dosed at 0.25 to 0.5 mg/kg per dose. Three doses per day is the usual maximum. Promethazine is available in tablets of 12.5, 25, and 50 mg, syrup of 6.25 and 25 mg per 5 ml, suppositories in 12.5, 25, and 50 mg strengths, and the injections in 25 and 50 mg/ml amps or vials. Flavored oral lozenges may be formulated by a compounding pharmacist.

TABLE *12.4.* Criteria for the Use of Prevention Medication.

1. The headaches interfere significantly with the child's functioning socially or at school. How much the headaches bother the child is a major consideration.
2. Failure of relaxation or biofeedback techniques. (These are only used after age 7 or 8.)
3. The child's and parents' willingness to utilize daily medication, with possible side effects.
4. Willingness of the child and parents to change medication, if necessary.
5. Failure of abortive medication to effectively treat the headaches.

TABLE 12.5. Quick Reference Guide: First Line Migraine and Tension Headache Prevention Medication in Children Under Age 11.

1. Cyproheptadine (Periactin): Cyproheptadine is a safe and generally effective first line headache preventive therapy. Fatigue and weight gain may be a problem, but it is usually well tolerated. Cyproheptadine is not as useful after age 11. It may be dosed once a day, and a convenient liquid form is available.
2. NSAIDs (ibuprofen, naproxen): Ibuprofen and naproxen are available as a liquid, and the lack of sedation renders these very helpful for daily use. GI side effects are relatively common, and when these are used on a long term basis, regular blood tests for hepatic and renal functions need to be done. Ibuprofen and naproxen may be utilized as daily preventives or as abortives for both tension and migraine headaches.
3. Propranolol (Inderal): Generally well tolerated, propranolol has been used for many years in children with migraine. Fatigue and decreased exercise tolerance may be a problem. With doses less than 60 mg per day, we need to use propranolol twice per day, which is inconvenient for most children. Cyproheptadine or NSAIDs should usually be prescribed prior to propranolol.

Preventive Medication for Migraine and CDH in Children Less Than 11 Years of Age

As stated earlier, the decision whether to use daily prevention medication for migraine or CDH depends upon many factors. If the migraines number three or four or more in a typical month, and are moderate or severe, prevention medication is indicated. However, if the child's migraines respond easily to an abortive, then I tend to simply use the abortive medication. Daily headaches that are more than mild usually warrant an attempt at preventive medication. Missed school time and the general effect of the headaches on the child's life need to be considered. Biofeedback and nonmedication therapies need to be introduced in any child over the age of 7 or 8 when headaches are severe.

In children younger than age 11, the preventive medications for migraine tend to be the same as the medications for chronic (tension) daily headache. The idea is always to use the minimum medication that is effective. First line medications for children include cyproheptadine (Periactin), NSAIDs (ibuprofen, naproxen), and propranolol (Inderal). Second line medications include amitriptyline (Elavil), and nortriptyline (Pamelor).

First Line Preventive Medication in Children Under Age 11

Cyproheptadine (Periactin)

Cyproheptadine is often the first choice for prevention; it is reasonably well tolerated but its effectiveness is somewhat limited. It is a safe medication, however. Side effects include fatigue and weight gain via increased appetite. These effects are common. The usual dosage is 4 to 12 mg per day. The tablets are scored, and there is also a liquid available (2 mg per 5 ml). I usually begin with 4 mg at night, and then increase to 6 or 8 mg at night. If this is not effective, the dose may be pushed to 12 mg total, usually 4 mg in the morning and 8 mg at night; 16 mg is unlikely to be more helpful than 12 mg. An alternative dosing schedule is 0.11 mg/lb per day.

Cyproheptadine is inexpensive, and the generic appears to be as effective as the brand name. It is available in 4 mg cyproheptadine or periactin tablets and as cyproheptadine syrup, 2 mg per 5 ml (teaspoon).

NSAIDs (Ibuprofen, Naproxen)

Anti-inflammatories will prevent headaches in both children and adults when taken daily. GI side effects are common, but serious renal or hepatic complications are very rare in children and adolescents. The lack of sedation or cognitive side effects are major advantages of the NSAIDs. Doses should be kept to a minimum, and regular blood tests need to be performed. The NSAIDs have been used for years for juvenile rheumatoid arthritis in doses much higher than we use with headache. For instance, with naproxen the daily dose for arthritis is 1 teaspoon twice a day at 55 lb (250 mg total), and 1.5 teaspoons twice a day at 84 lb (375 mg per day). Doses for headache are half of this (or less).

For daily use, the usual dose of ibuprofen at age 5 is $\frac{1}{2}$ teaspoon of the 100 mg per teaspoon syrup, or 50 mg per day. At ages 6 to 8, the dose is $\frac{1}{2}$ to 1 teaspoon, or 50 to 100 mg per day. At ages 9 to 10, the dose increases to 1 or 2 teaspoons, or 100 to 200 mg per day. At 200 mg per day, one pill of the 200 mg ibuprofen may be used.

With naproxen, the dose at 40 to 55 lb is $\frac{1}{2}$ teaspoon daily (approximately 62 mg). At 55 to 85 lb, it is $\frac{1}{2}$ or 1 teaspoon daily (62 to 125 mg). One teaspoon is equal to one half of the 250 mg pill, and some children may be able to swallow one half of the naprosyn pill. Above 85 lb, the dose increases to 1 to 2 teaspoons. At 2 teaspoons, the whole 250 mg pill is equivalent. As with any medication, we strive to attain the smallest possible dose of the anti-inflammatories. For more information on ibuprofen and naproxen, see above sections on abortive therapy.

Propranolol (Inderal)

For many years, propranolol has been a mainstay of headache preventive therapy. The side effects are usually minimal in children. Propranolol is effective in migraine, and occasionally for daily headache. However, because of the possible decrease in heart rate and blood pressure, with a corresponding decrease in exercise tolerance, I use cyproheptadine or NSAIDs more often than propranolol. The usual dose of propranolol is 1 to 4 mg/kg/day, either in two doses or with one long acting capsule. I usually begin with 10 mg twice per day, and titrate up to 40 or 60 mg per day. With most children, I do not exceed 80 mg per day, but doses much higher have been used. One disadvantage of propranolol over most other beta blockers is that the once a day capsules cannot be divided. With nadolol (Corgard), for example, the pills are scored, rendering dosage adjustments much easier.

Side effects of propranolol are usually minimal in children. Fatigue and GI (usually lower abdominal) upset are relatively common. Weight gain is more common in adults. Propranolol cannot be used if the child has asthma, and if the child becomes short of breath the drug needs to be stopped. Cognitive side effects, such as memory or concentration difficulties, may occur. Dizziness or lightheadedness may be seen at times. Propranolol is available in tablets of 10, 20, 40, 60, 80, and 90 mg. The long acting capsules (propranolol or Inderal LA) are available in 60, 80, 120, and 160 mg. Propranolol is also discussed in Chapter 3.

Second Line Preventive Medications in Children Under Age 11

After cyproheptadine, NSAIDs, and propranolol have been tried, the antidepressants may be used. In children with moderate or severe CDH (Chronic Daily Headache), the antidepressants may be utilized as a first line therapy. Amitriptyline (Elavil) and nortriptyline (Pamelor, Aventyl) have been widely used in children and adolescents, and are generally well tolerated. Antidepressants help headaches not because the patients are depressed, but because of a more direct antiheadache effect, mediated primarily through serotonergic mechanisms.

Amitriptyline and nortriptyline are very similar. Amitriptyline is somewhat more effective, but nortriptyline has less side effects. With both amitriptyline and nortriptyline, the dose is initiated at 10 mg each night, and increased, if necessary, to 25 or 50 mg. Occasionally, I will push the dose to 75 or 100 mg, but the average dose in this age range is 25 mg. The medications are usually given at night. However, at times, daytime dosing may be more effective. Nortriptyline is available in a liquid form, which is occasionally helpful in children.

Side effects include fatigue, anxiety, weight gain, dry mouth, and dizziness. Memory or concentration difficulties may ensue. Tachycardia may be a problem, and blurred vision is occasionally a concern. Although sedation is common, insomnia may also occur. The anticholinergic side effects are somewhat less with nortriptyline. Amitriptyline (Elavil) is available in tablets of 10, 25, 50, 75, 100, and 150 mg. Nortriptyline (Pamelor) is available in capsules of 10, 25, 50, and 75 mg. The liquid is available as a 10 mg per 5 ml (teaspoon) solution that contains 4% alcohol. For a more complete discussion of amitriptyline and nortriptyline, see Chapters 3 and 7.

Abortive Medication for Adolescents 11 Years and Older

Much of the previous discussion of medications for children also applies to adolescents. However, in adolescents, the medication regimens begin to resemble those that we use for adults. As always, medication is kept to a minimum, and alternative methods of treatment, such as biofeedback or relaxation therapies, are encouraged. As much as we try to encourage and push biofeedback and, at times, counseling, we are usually left with medication as the primary treatment for the adolescent.

Most adolescents do not require daily preventive medication for their headaches, and we attempt to simply use abortive medication. However, at times the headaches are severe or frequent, and daily preventive medication is necessary. It is usually an easy choice as to whether to utilize daily preventive medication. Occasionally, the number and severity of headaches places the patient in the borderline or gray zone. At this point, the efficacy of the abortive medication with that patient plays a crucial role in determining whether to proceed with a preventive approach. If a simple abortive medication eliminates the headache with minimal side effects, we can forego daily preventive therapy. The input of the family always plays an important role in medication decisions. As with all age groups, I try and wean adolescents off of daily medications periodically, to assess whether the headaches have naturally improved.

Tension Headache Abortive Medication in Adolescents

In treating tension headaches, we never want to "chase" after the headache all day with abortive medication. If patients need to do this, we avoid the rebound headache situation by utilizing preventive medication. There is a staggering array of preventive medications available for tension headache. Generally, nonaddicting medications are used for this type of headache. For more information on tension headache, see Chapter 6.

The first line tension headache abortive medications for adolescents are: acetaminophen, ibuprofen, naproxen, aspirin, Aspirin Free Excedrin, Anacin, Excedrin, and Norgesic Forte. Second line abortives include Midrin and the butalbital compounds (Fiorinal, Esgic, Phrenilin).

First Line Tension Headache Abortive Medications

Acetaminophen

Acetaminophen is very well tolerated and is the usual first choice for tension headache. It is not as effective as the NSAIDs or aspirin, but has less side effects. Adding caffeine, such as a soft drink, may enhance the effectiveness. Aspirin Free Excedrin contains acetaminophen plus caffeine. The usual dose is 325 to 650 mg every 4 to 6 hours, as needed. For a complete discussion of acetaminophen, and forms available, see above section on acetaminophen in the discussion on children under 11 years.

Ibuprofen

Ibuprofen and the anti-inflammatories are more effective than acetaminophen for headache, but these drugs have more side effects. GI upset is fairly common, and if any of the NSAIDs are used frequently, blood tests need to be periodically monitored for renal and hepatic functions. The usual dose for ibuprofen is 200 or 400 mg every 4 to 6 hours, as needed. There is a liquid ibuprofen available (Children's Advil, 100 mg per 5 cc). For other available forms, see above section on ibuprofen.

Naproxen (Naprosyn, Anaprox)

Naproxen is widely utilized as an abortive medication for adolescents and adults; at times, it may be effective when ibuprofen is not helpful. GI upset is common, and with frequent use blood tests need to be monitored for liver and kidney functions. The NSAIDs should be taken with something to eat in order to buffer the stomach. The usual dose is one Naprosyn 250 mg pill or one Anaprox 275 mg pill every 4 hours, as needed. This dose may be increased in older adolescents to a 375 or 500 mg Naprosyn, or one 550 mg Anaprox DS, not to exceed two in 1 day. The Naprosyn tablets are scored, rendering dosage adjustments very easy. There is a liquid Naprosyn, 125 mg per 5 cc. Anaprox, which is naproxen sodium, may be more effective for abortive therapy than naproxen (Naprosyn) itself. Available forms include Anaprox tablets, 275 mg (250 mg naproxen base), Anaprox DS, 550 mg (500 mg naproxen base), and Naprosyn tablets of 250, 375, and 500 mg. The liquid Naprosyn is available as an oral suspension, 125 mg per 5 ml (teaspoon). For further discussion of naproxen, see Chapters 2, 3, and 6.

Aspirin

Aspirin is the old, reliable, standard headache medication. Because of the concern over Reyes' syndrome, it has decreased in popularity, but should not be excluded as a headache abortive. Due to the possibility of Reyes' syndrome, aspirin should not be used in children and adolescents who have varicella or influenza infections, but otherwise may be used for headache relief. GI upset is common, but aspirin is generally well tolerated. Caffeine, such as in soft drinks, may enhance the efficacy. The usual dose is 325 mg every 4 to 6 hours, as needed. Aspirin with caffeine compounds (Anacin, Excedrin) are discussed further in this chapter. Smaller doses need to be used in children.

Aspirin Free Excedrin

This is a useful combination of 250 mg of acetaminophen and 65 mg of caffeine. The caffeine enhances the effectiveness of the acetaminophen, and this combination is well tolerated. The caffeine may cause nervousness or insomnia. This combination should not be overused, because rebound headaches from overuse of caffeine may ensue. The usual dose is one tablet every 4 to 6 hours, as needed.

Anacin

Anacin contains 400 mg of aspirin, and 32 mg of caffeine, without acetaminophen. Anacin is more effective than Aspirin Free Excedrin because aspirin is more effective than acetaminophen. Anacin has less caffeine than Excedrin E.S. and thus, although less effective, leads to fewer rebound headaches. Since there is concern about long term renal effects of aspirin, caffeine, and acetaminophen combinations, Anacin should be used prior to Excedrin if we are anticipating long term use.

GI side effects are common, and nervousness may occur because of the caffeine. The usual dose is one Anacin every 4 to 6 hours, as needed. Forms available are Anacin and Anacin Maximum Strength (500 mg of aspirin and 32 mg of caffeine).

Extra Strength Excedrin

These tablets contain 250 mg of acetaminophen, 250 mg of aspirin, and 65 mg of caffeine. The extra caffeine, 65 mg versus 32 mg in Anacin, adds to efficacy but also increases side effects. Rebound headaches are somewhat more likely to occur with Excedrin. There is concern about the long term renal effects of the combination of aspirin, caffeine, and acetaminophen. However, many adolescents and adults find Excedrin to be one of the most effective OTC preparations. There are many other similar preparations, but Excedrin is the best known of these drugs.

GI side effects are common, as is nervousness due to the caffeine. The usual dose is one tablet every 4 to 6 hours, as needed.

Norgesic Forte

Norgesic Forte contains a combination of aspirin, 770 mg, caffeine, 60 mg, and orphenadrine citrate, 50 mg. The orphenadrine is an antihistamine with muscle relaxant properties. This is a strong combination of medications, but is not addicting. Because of the large amount of aspirin, the usual dose is one half of a pill every 3 to 4 hours, as needed. One whole pill may be used, if tolerated.

GI side effects are common, and nervousness may occur due to the caffeine. The orphenadrine may cause drowsiness. In addition, anticholinergic side effects, such as dry mouth or blurred vision, may occur because of the orphenadrine. (See Chapter 2.)

Second Line Tension Headache Abortives in Adolescents

If the above medications are not helpful, I usually use Midrin, which is primarily a migraine abortive, or the butalbital compounds, which are habit forming. These include Fiorinal, Fioricet, Esgic, and Phrenilin. All of these butalbital compounds differ slightly in composition. These need to be limited per day and per month in all patients. Midrin is extensively discussed in the above section on migraine abortive medications in children, and in Chapter 2. Butalbital compounds are discussed in Chapter 2, and in the above section on migraine abortive medications for children.

Migraine Abortive Therapy in Adolescents

The vast majority of migraine patients do not require daily preventive medication. We rely on abortive medication to ease the pain and shorten the duration of the migraine. For many adolescents, Aspirin Free Excedrin or Extra Strength Excedrin is all that is needed. Ibuprofen, naproxen, Midrin, Norgesic Forte, and the butalbital compounds are all useful at times. Ergots are effective, but have increased side effects. Antinausea medication is very helpful for many patients. DHE, as a nasal spray or injection, is utilized in this age range, but sumatripton currently is not. Abortive therapy is discussed in Chapter 2, and previously in this chapter.

Preventive Therapy in Adolescents

Chronic Daily Headache Preventive Therapy in Adolescents

Many adolescents are plagued by daily headaches, as well as migraines. Depression may be present in these patients, and this needs to be addressed. However, psychotherapy and/or biofeedback are not appropriate for some adolescents and not effective in others. Many of these patients, as with adults, need some type of daily preventive medications for the moderate or severe headaches. Taking a biological viewpoint of daily "tension" headaches (CDH) is a more realistic approach than looking at these headaches as a psychological problem.

When daily headaches are present, and are moderate or severe, we do not want to "chase" after the pain all day with abortive medications. We often simply create rebound headaches by doing this. The preventive medications for CDH include anti-inflammatories, antidepressants, and

---

TABLE 12.6. Quick Reference Guide: Prevention Medication for Chronic Daily Headache in Adolescents.

First Line Therapy

1. NSAIDs: Frequent GI upset is seen, but the NSAIDs usually do not cause fatigue or other cognitive effects. Ibuprofen (Motrin) and naproxen (Naprosyn, Anaprox) are the NSAIDs most frequently utilized. Liquid preparations are available for both of these. Doses need to be kept to a minimum; hepatic and renal functions should be monitored via regular blood tests.

Second Line Therapy

1. Antidepressants: Highly effective for daily headache; these are often effective for migraine as well as daily headache. Nortriptyline (Pamelor, Aventyl), protriptyline (Vivactil) and amitriptyline (Elavil) are most commonly used. Usually well tolerated in low doses, and safe for long term use. Cognitive side effects, dry mouth, and dizziness are common.
2. Beta blockers: Occasionally effective for daily headache, but generally more useful with migraine. Propranolol (Inderal) and nadolol (Corgard) are most commonly utilized. Beta blockers may decrease exercise tolerance, which is a problem in this age range. Cognitive side effects also limit the utility of beta blockers.

---

beta blackers. As with adults, the antidepressants tend to be the most effective medications, not because they are helping depression, but because they directly affect the headaches through serotonergic pathways. However, anti-inflammatories are preferred for first line treatment because they are well tolerated in this age group. If the anti-inflammatories are not effective, we progress on to the antidepressants or beta blockers. (See also Chapter 7 and the above section on preventive therapy for children.)

First Line Preventive Therapy for CDH in Adolescents

The anti-inflammatories should usually be used prior to other medications, because of the lack of sedation and CNS side effects. They are generally well tolerated, but regular blood tests for renal and hepatic functions need to be performed. GI side effects are common, and these medications should be taken with food.

Ibuprofen and naproxen are the primary anti-inflammatories. They are discussed extensively in Chapter 2, and in the above section on abortive medications for children. The usual dose of ibuprofen in adolescents is 200 to 400 mg per day. Liquid Advil is available for those who do not like to swallow pills. Naproxen is usually used at 250 to 500 mg of Naprosyn per day, in one dose. Alternatively, one Anaprox, 275 mg, or one Anaprox D.S., 550 mg, may be taken each day.

TABLE 12.7. Quick Reference Guide: First Line Migraine Preventive Medication for Adolescents.

1. Anti-inflammatories: Frequent GI upset is seen, but the NSAIDs usually do not cause fatigue or other cognitive effects. Ibuprofen (Motrin) and naproxen (Naprosyn, Anaprox) are the NSAIDs most frequently utilized. Liquid preparations are available for both of these. Doses need to be kept to a minimum; hepatic and renal functions should be monitored via regular blood tests.
2. Verapamil (Isoptin, Calan, Veralan): A calcium antagonist, effective for migraine, and occasionally, daily headache. Generally well tolerated, with constipation common. Convenient once per day dosing with the sustained release form.
3. Antidepressants: Highly effective for migraine and daily headache. Nortriptyline (Pamelor, Aventyl), protriptyline (Vivactil), and amitriptyline (Elavil) are most commonly used. Usually well tolerated in low doses and safe for long term use. Cognitive side effects, dry mouth, and dizziness are common.
4. Beta blockers: Effective for migraine, and occasionally for daily headache. Propranolol (Inderal) and nadolol (Corgard) are most commonly utilized. Beta blockers may decrease exercise tolerance, which is a problem in this age range. Cognitive side effects also limit the utility of beta blockers.

Second Line Preventive Medication for CDH in Adolescents

The antidepressants and beta blockers are the preventive medications to institute if naproxen or ibuprofen are not helpful. Antidepressants are, in general, the most successful medications for daily headaches. Antidepressants are extensively discussed in Chapters 3 and 7.

The antidepressants most often used in this age group include protriptyline (Vivactil), amitriptyline (Elavil), and nortriptyline (Pamelor, Aventyl). Please refer to Chapter 7 for a discussion of these medications. Protriptyline is a very useful drug in this age group because of its lack of sedation or weight gain side effects. Amitriptyline is inexpensive and very effective, both for migraine and daily headache. Sedation is very common with amitriptyline. Nortriptyline is a milder version of amitriptyline, with less efficacy but decreased side effects. Nortriptyline is well tolerated, and useful for all ages.

The usual beta blockers used for daily headaches are propranolol (Inderal) and nadolol (Corgard). These are generally more effective in migraine prophylaxis, but some patients with daily headaches respond very well to the beta blockers. Antidepressants are generally more effective for daily headaches, however. Sedation and decreased exercise tolerance are common side effects. Lower abdominal upset may occur. Beta blockers are discussed at length in Chapters 3, and in the above section on prevention medication for children.

Migraine Preventive Therapy in Adolescents

When migraines occur more than four times per month, or are very severe, preventive therapy is usually very helpful. Two very severe headaches per month, with nausea, are very upsetting to one's life, and the anticipation of the headache adds to the problem. Thus, at times we will institute daily medication for as little as one or two very severe migraines per month. The goal, as always, is to decrease frequency or severity by at least 70% with as little medication as possible.

The first line migraine preventive medications for adolescents are anti-inflammatories, beta blockers, the calcium blocker verapamil, and tricyclic antidepressants. Because of a favorable side effect profile, the anti-inflammatories are utilized first. It these are not effective, the beta blockers or antidepressants or verapamil may be used. These have all been discussed previously in the above sections and in Chapter 3.

The second line migraine prevention medications include valproate (Depakote) and fluoxetine (Prozac). Depakote is discussed in Chapter 3. It is generally effective in migraine. Side effects and the need for frequent blood tests limit the use of Depakote. Prozac has been helpful for many adult patients with migraine, but its use in younger age ranges has been limited. However, it is helpful at times in older adolescents with migraine and daily headaches. See Chapters 3 and 7 for a discussion of Prozac.

The third line migraine prevention medications in this age group include phenelzine (Nardil), an MAO inhibitor, and IV DHE therapy. These are discussed in Chapter 3. Phenelzine, although effective in migraine and daily headache, should only be reserved for the most refractive situations, because of the risk of a hypertensive crisis. The physician needs to absolutely trust the patient to follow the diet and avoid certain medications while on phenelzine. IV DHE, given in the office or at the hospital for four to nine doses, will often alleviate headaches for a period of time. IV DHE is discussed earlier in this chapter, and in Chapter 3.

CHAPTER 13

Special Headache Topics

In this chapter, the following six headache topics are discussed: (1) treatment of headache after age 50, (2) post-traumatic headache, (3) occipital nerve injections for neuralgia and unilateral headache syndromes, (4) indomethacin responsive unilateral headaches (chronic paroxysmal hemicrania and hemicrania continua), (5) exertional and sexual headache, and (6) lumbar puncture headache.

Headache After Age 50

Although it is true that the incidence of migraine, cluster, and tension headache decreases after age 50, headache continues to be a major problem for many people. The vast majority of patients with headaches after age 50 have had preexisting migraine, tension, or cluster headache, but a significant number of people begin suffering from headache in their 50s or 60s.

When headache begins de novo in adults, a workup is usually indicated, and this is particularly true with advancing age. Intracranial pathology, giant cell arteritis, thrombotic cerebrovascular disease, meningitis, and hypertension need to be excluded. In addition, cervical spine disorders may play a role in producing headache in this population. Systemic disease, such as chronic renal disease, anemia, and respiratory disorders, contribute to headache. The effect of various medications needs to be considered.

The presence of focal neurologic symptoms requires investigation. A workup is indicated when preexisting headache patterns change dramatically. It is a very difficult situation in patients with a long history of migraine who have had an MRI scan in the past, and now develop new intracranial pathology. The pathology may go undetected because we do not usually continue to scan headache patients every year.

Cervical spine disease may contribute to headache. However, this is generally overdiagnosed, as cervical radiologic changes are very common after age 50. Headache of cervical origin is usually occipital in location and is often described as a dull ache. However, tension headache may occur in this location, and it may be difficult to differentiate between the two conditions. Unfortunately, treatment directed at the cervical spine usually leads to less than satisfactory results. Although physical therapy and anti-inflammatories may help, they are often disappointing.

Patients may experience migraine aura without the headache. These auras need to be distinguished from transient ischemic attacks. Depression may exacerbate headache, and the antidepressants often decrease both the headache and depression. However, the mechanism of action of antidepressants for headache is usually independent of the antidepressant effect.

The primary headache types after age 50 or 60 are the same as in younger ages; migraine, tension, and cluster. The principles of treatment, as outlined in previous chapters, remain the same; however, in an older population, our medication choices are somewhat limited. Anti-inflammatories are used less often because of increased renal and GI toxicity. We use lesser doses with many medications. Ergotamines, with the exception of DHE-45, are generally not employed. Sumatriptan (Imitrex) injections have been valuable in patients under age 65.

Migraine Headache after Age 50

The general principles for utilizing migraine preventives and abortives are the same in this age range as for younger patients, as discussed in Chapters 2 and 3. Nonmedication instructions such as diet, maintaining regular sleeping patterns, placing ice to the pain, etc., remain valid, but biofeedback or relaxation techniques are significantly less useful in older patients.

First Line Migraine Prevention Medication in the Elderly

The first line preventive medications are similar to those in younger age ranges, with one exception: naproxen is utilized less often in older patients. For abortive therapy, the anti-inflammatories are helpful at all ages, but I attempt to avoid the daily use of anti-inflammatories in older patients. Amitriptyline, propranolol, and verapamil are the first line migraine preventives. Antidepressants other than amitriptyline may be helpful. These include, among others, nortriptyline (Pamelor, Aventyl) and fluoxetine (Prozac). Antidepressants are particularly beneficial for daily headaches. Fluoxetine is generally well tolerated. In addition to propranolol, many other beta blockers are useful, such as nadolol, atenolol, or metoprolol. The above medications are discussed at length in Chapters 3 and 7.

Second and Third Line Migraine Preventive Strategies in the Elderly

Second line therapies include polypharmacy (combining two of the first line medications) and Depakote. Methysergide (Sansert) is a helpful second line medication in younger age ranges, but is not usually utilized after age 50.

Third line strategies include MAO inhibitors, such as phenelzine, and repetitive IV DHE injections. Both of these regimens are used with great caution in older patients. In addition, NSAIDs are considered a third line approach in this age range. These medications are discussed at length in Chapter 3.

Migraine Abortive Medication in the Elderly

Cold packs about the head, a dark and quiet room, and sleep remain mainstays of abortive therapy for migraine. However, patients usually require medication. After age 50, the ergotamines, except for DHE, are rarely utilized. The usual abortive medications include caffeine, Extra Strength Excedrin, naproxen (Naprosyn or Anaprox), ibuprofen, ketorolac, Midrin, Norgesic Forte, butalbital compounds (Fiorinal, Fioricet, Esgic, Phrenilin, Fiorinal with codeine), DHE injections (IM) or nasal spray, sumatriptan injections (Imitrex), corticosteroids, narcotics, and sedatives. These are extensively discussed in Chapter 2. Antiemetic medications are very helpful for many patients, and these are also described in Chapter 2.

The choice of abortive medication depends upon many factors, such as concurrent medical conditions, the presence of nausea, and the age of the patient. DHE and sumatriptan are not used after age 65. If the patient has significant cardiac risk factors, or uncontrolled HTN, I hesitate to utilize DHE or sumatriptan. The anti-inflammatories are used with caution in the elderly. After age 75 or 80, I often prescribe one half of a pill of a milder narcotic preparation, such as hydrocodone, thus avoiding NSAIDs or aspirin. Among the butalbital compounds, Phrenilin is used more often with increasing age, primarily because it does not contain aspirin or caffeine.

Tension Headache after Age 50

Tension headache is common in all ages, and is extensively discussed in Chapters 6 and 7. Tension headache is an unfortunate choice of terms because it implies that tension in the patient's life is at the root of the headache; stress and tension may exacerbate an underlying primary headache disorder, but are not usually their cause. The vast majority of patients with daily headache also suffer from migraine. After age 50, migraines often diminish, leaving a chronic daily headache (CDH).

TABLE 13.1. Quick Reference Guide: Migraine Preventive Therapy in the Elderly.

First Line Therapy

1. Amitriptyline: Effective, inexpensive, also helpful for daily headaches and insomnia. Use in very low doses, all at night. Sedation, weight gain, dry mouth, constipation, and tachycardia are common. Initial dose is 10 mg, which may even be cut in half to 5 mg, working up to 25 or 50 mg; may be pushed to 100 or 150 mg.
2. Propranolol: Effective; long acting capsules may be dosed once a day. Occasionally useful for daily headaches. Sedation, diarrhea, GI upset, and weight gain are common. Very useful in combination with amitriptyline. Begin with the long acting 60 mg capsule once per day. Average dose is 60 to 120 mg per day (dose may be increased in younger age ranges).
3. Verapamil: Reasonably effective for migraine, convenient once per day dosing with the slow release (SR) tablets. Usually nonsedating, and weight gain is uncommon. Occasionally helpful for daily headaches. May be combined with other first line medications, particularly amitriptyline. Constipation is common. Starting dose is one half of a 180 or 240 mg SR pill, increasing quickly to one per day. May be pushed to 240 mg twice a day, or decreased to as little as one half of a 180 mg SR tablet each day.

Second Line Therapy

1. Polypharmacy: The combination of two preventives is often more effective than one drug. Amitriptyline may be combined with propranolol, particularly if the tachycardia of the amitriptyline needs to be offset by a beta blocker. This combination is the most commonly used one for "mixed" headaches (migraine plus CDH).
2. Valproate (Depakote): This seizure medication is becoming increasingly popular for migraine prevention. Liver functions need to be monitored in the beginning of treatment. Common side effects include lethargy, GI upset, cognitive effects, weight gain, and alopecia. Dosage varies from 250 to 2,000 mg per day, in divided doses. The average dose is 1,000 mg per day. On the higher doses, levels need to be checked for toxicity.

Third Line Therapy

1. Phenelzine (Nardil): An MAO inhibitor, phenelzine is a powerful migraine and daily headache preventive medication. Phenelzine may be used alone, or in combination with amitriptyline, verapamil, or propranolol. Phenelzine is very helpful for depression, anxiety, and panic attacks. The risk of a hypertensive crisis is small but is a major drawback to this type of medication. Dietary restrictions render MAO inhibitors difficult for the patient. Side effects include insomnia, weight gain, dry mouth, and constipation. The usual dose is 45 mg each night (3 of the 15 mg tablets). This can be adjusted up or down, and the average range is from one to five tablets per day.
2. Repetitive IV DHE therapy: DHE should be used with caution in patients over the age of 50, as coronary artery spasm, although very rare, may occur. Helpful for patients with frequent or status migraine, this therapy often provides weeks or months of headache improvement. IV DHE can be done in the office or hospital. Side effects include nausea, a feeling of warmth about the head, leg cramps, or diarrhea. In the office, the protocol consists of a pill of metoclopramide (10 mg), followed in $\frac{1}{2}$ hour by the DHE. For the first dose, $\frac{1}{2}$ mg is given, and, if well tolerated, the subsequent doses are 1 mg. Three or four doses are given in the office, and up to nine doses in the hospital. After the IV DHE, migraine prevention medication is usually instituted. This protocol is discussed in Chapter 3.
3. NSAIDs: Anti-inflammatories, such as naproxen, ibuprofen, and flurbiprofen, are discussed in Chapters 2, 3, and 6. I utilize these in older patients only as a third line approach because of increased GI and renal effects. However, in certain patients the NSAIDs are effective for migraine and daily headache. When utilized daily, frequent blood tests need to be performed.

There are two categories of tension headache: episodic tension headache, and chronic tension headache (CDH). The "as needed" abortive therapy is essentially the same for the two types. When chronic daily tension-type headache is moderate or severe, the preventive medication approach becomes very important. It is possible that tension-type headache has an underlying pathophysiology similar to migraine, and that we are observing different parts of a spectrum. It is clear that people are predisposed to these headaches, and they are not a "psychological" problem. Stress does affect tension headaches, as it does most illnesses. Strategies for coping with psychological factors in headache patients are discussed in Chapter 1.

The decision to utilize preventive medication depends upon whether the daily headaches are mild, moderate, or severe. Daily pain medications need to be kept to a minimum, to avoid the rebound headache situation.

For patients with episodic tension headaches, the abortive medication approach is usually all that is necessary. However, if patients overuse analgesic medication, preventive therapy may be beneficial. For abortive treatment of episodic tension headaches, see Chapter 6.

Chronic Daily Headache

When tension headaches are daily or almost daily, analgesics are often consumed in excessive amounts, thus creating rebound headaches. Many patients take large numbers of OTC medications, resulting in increased headaches.

For CDH that is moderate or severe and interferes with the quality of life, the preventive medication approach is utilized. Stress management, psychological counseling, or relaxation strategies do have a role to play in certain patients, and should be offered as a treatment option. Most patients experiencing moderate or severe daily headaches will benefit from a preventive medication approach.

First Line Preventive Therapy for CDH

The antidepressants are the mainstay of therapy for daily headaches. They are effective whether or not the patient is depressed, and the reason that they benefit headaches is usually independent of antidepressant action. The choice of antidepressant depends upon many factors, including the anxiety level of the patient, presence of a sleep disturbance, age of the patient, and other medical conditions. If the patient has a tendency towards constipation, that also will influence our choice.

There are many antidepressants from which to choose, and not all are effective for headaches. The tricyclic antidepressants have been the most widely utilized and are very effective. Fluoxetine (Prozac) is gaining acceptance as a first line daily headache preventive. Sertraline (Zoloft) is a serotonin reuptake inhibitor similar to Prozac. Zoloft is well tolerated and is effective for certain patients. The most commonly used medication for daily headaches is amitriptyline. In the elderly population, nortriptyline (Pamelor) is generally preferred over amitriptyline because of the milder anticholinergic and sedative effects. However, nortriptyline is less effective. Fluoxetine (Prozac) is often a good choice, as is desipramine (Norpramin), because of decreased side effects. For a complete discussion of the above, see Chapters 3 and 7.

Second line daily preventive medications include valproate (Depakote), beta blockers such as propranolol, muscle relaxants, and calcium blockers (verapamil). The NSAIDs are not a first or second line preventive therapy after age 50 or 60, because of increased renal and GI toxicity. Third line prevention therapy includes MAO inhibitors (phenelzine), NSAIDs, or polypharmacy (combining, for instance, an antidepressant and a beta blocker). All of the above are discussed in detail in Chapters 3 and 7.

Cluster Headache after Age 50

The treatment of cluster headache after age 50 is, in most respects, the same as the treatment of cluster in younger patients. Most patients have episodic cluster headaches and do not need medication except when they are in a cluster series. Chronic cluster sufferers, of course, require constant therapy. With most cluster patients, there is a need for daily preventive medication and abortive medicine. Cluster headaches are also discussed in Chapters 9, 10, and 11.

Preventive Therapy for Cluster Headache

The primary preventive medications remain the same: verapamil (Calan, Isoptin), lithium, and corticosteroids. Corticosteroids should be minimized, and generally used in low doses, saving them for the "peak" of the cluster period. Episodic cluster periods often slowly increase in intensity over days to weeks, and they then peak in intensity. With chronic cluster, patients also experience peaks throughout the year, and small amounts of corticosteroids may be utilized at these times. Verapamil and/or lithium remain the standard cluster preventives, and these are usually well tolerated in the older patient. Sansert, which is only minimally helpful in most cluster patients, should not usually be employed in this age range.

Valproate (Depakote) is a recent addition to the armamentarium. Valproate should be considered after corticosteroids, lithium, and verapamil. It is usually well tolerated, but blood tests need to be monitored. IV DHE is a strong consideration as a second line preventive medication and may be administered in the office as a course of four injections over 2 days. The IV DHE will often help for a period of time until the preventive medication takes effect. Occipital injections of corticosteroids, such as betamethasone or Depo-Medrol, are effective and well tolerated. These injections usually give 1 to 2 weeks of relief. In patients with refractive chronic cluster, radiofrequency gangliorhizolysis is a reasonable alternative to medication. For a complete discussion of cluster preventive therapy, see Chapter 10.

Abortive Therapy for Cluster Headache

The abortive approach differs slightly for older age ranges, as we use less ergotamines (except DHE). Oxygen remains a mainstay of therapy, and should be tried in all patients. Ice packs are utilized directly where the pain is most severe. Pain medications have relatively little use, for by the time they may take effect, most cluster episodes have ceased. However, the pain of cluster is often so severe that the anticipation of the cluster becomes a major problem; patients find comfort knowing that they possess an analgesic that may dampen the intense pain. Lidocaine nose spray may help to a small degree, and is very well tolerated. DHE injections are often helpful, but need to be used with caution in patients with risk factors for coronary artery disease. Sumatriptan injections are extremely effective for cluster headache, and may be used up to age 65. Sumatriptan is generally better tolerated than DHE. With the use of DHE or sumatriptan, chest pain or pressure may occur.

The standard ergotamines, such as sublingual ergotamine (Ergostat), must be used with great caution after age 50 because of coronary artery constriction. It is important to minimize the dose of ergotamine, by using one half of an Ergostat tablet (the tablet is 2 mg) or one third to one half of a Cafergot suppository. The pills of Cafergot are not usually effective, because of the delayed onset of action.

Pain medications include butalbital compounds (Fiorinal, Fiorinal with codeine, Fioricet, Esgic, Phrenilin), and narcotics or sedatives. These are helpful for lengthy clusters. In general, analgesics are not extremely effective for cluster headache, but it is often helpful for patients to know that an analgesic is available. In the emergency room, as a last resort for a long, severe cluster headache, intramuscular narcotics are occasionally useful. This situation occurs during the peak of the cluster period. Overuse of narcotics, and possible addiction, is a potential problem with cluster patients, primarily because of the intense, horrible pain. For a complete discussion of abortive therapy for cluster headache, see Chapter 9.

Post-traumatic Headache

The post-traumatic headache syndrome is a very common sequelae following injuries to the head or neck, and often occurs after rear-end auto accidents. The headaches are usually self-limited and resolve quickly, within days to several weeks. The vast majority of patients with post-traumatic headaches simply want their pain to be improved and their disrupted life back to normal. Surprisingly few are malingering or exaggerating their symptoms.

In many patients, particularly those with more severe trauma, headaches may be a problem for months, years, or a lifetime. If the headaches develop within 2 weeks of the event, and persist for more than several months, we would consider this to be the chronic phase of the post-traumatic headache syndrome. Occasionally, patients do not develop post-traumatic migraines until months following the injury, but headaches usually begin within hours or days of the accident.

Predicting which patients will continue to suffer chronic, unremitting post-traumatic pain is a difficult undertaking. In general, patients with a preexisting headache or migraine problem are at increased risk. Patients with a strong family history of migraine may be at increased risk for developing chronic headaches. Severity of trauma may also aid in predicting outcome, but many patients endure months or years of severe headaches after trivial head trauma. Rear-end auto collisions, without head trauma, commonly produce severe headaches and cervical pain. Factors such as the angle of impact, where the patient was sitting in the car, and what happened to the brain within the skull are key elements in producing the headaches.

Many patients have associated neck and posterior occipital pain. The neck pain tends to be independent of the headaches, and the cervical pain and headaches may resolve at different times. Physical therapy is a key element in treating the associated neck pain and tenderness, and physical therapy may also decrease the headaches.

The headaches are usually of two types: (1) tension-type headache that may be daily or episodic, and (2) migraine headaches that are usually more severe. In some patients, the post-traumatic migraine headaches are the major problem, with a periodic severe headache lasting hours to days. In other patients, the tension-type headache is the predominant problem. Many post-traumatic patients have mixed headaches, with both CDH and migraines. The occipital aching pain, so often associated with the neck pain, is usually considered to be of muscular origin. However, the occipital pain may respond to therapies for cervical pain, and at other times the occipital pain improves with the standard tension headache medications.

Medical work-up for post-traumatic headaches includes, if necessary, a CAT or an MRI scan to rule out an intracranial hemorrhage. There is also consideration for performing an EEG. The work-up is usually limited and is done according to the physician's clinical judgement. Most patients with mild post-traumatic headaches do not need to undergo extensive testing other than a neurologic exam.

There are many other symptoms that often accompany the post-traumatic headache syndrome. These tend to be similar in most patients. They include some or all of the following: poor concentration, becoming easily angered, sensitivity to noise or bright lights, depression, dizziness or vertigo, tinnitus, memory problems, fatigue, insomnia, lack of motivation, decreased libido, nervousness or anxiety, irritability, becoming easily frustrated, and decreased ability to comprehend complex issues.

The presence of headaches, neck pain, and the symptoms in the above paragraph often lead physicians, coworkers, and family members to conclude that the patient is exaggerating the complaints. However, in the vast majority of post-traumatic patients, every complaint is real, not exaggerated, and these people simply wish to feel better. The post-traumatic headache syndrome ranges from mild to severe and is often disabling to a person's life. Most patients have some degree of difficulty with their home or work life because of the headaches, anxiety, insomnia, and concentration difficulties. It then becomes a vicious cycle, with more psychological stress being placed on the patient because of the difficulties at work and at home. Unfortunately, our legal and insurance processes are not entirely fair to many of these patients, because objective testing does not reveal deficits in the vast majority of these injured patients. They are often unfairly viewed as functional or malingering.

As mentioned above, accompanying the post-traumatic headache problem is the very frequent neck pain. This is usually secondary to soft tissue damage to ligaments and muscles, but may involve disc damage and, occasionally, nerve root compression as well. Sensitivity over the occipital nerve area is very common and occipital neuralgia may accompany the post-traumatic headaches. We frequently find trigger points in the trapezius, posterior cervical, and occipital areas, with muscle spasm in these areas being very common. It is not infrequent to find such severe spasm that patients have almost zero range of motion of their cervical spine, and the neck muscles feel extremely tight upon palpation.

Treatment of the post-traumatic syndrome involves one or several of the following: medication, physical therapy, psychological counseling, and relaxation training/biofeedback. Most patients do not need all of the modalities of therapy, and treatment programs need to be individualized. First and foremost, reassurance that this condition will improve is important, as in the vast majority of cases, the headaches and neck pain progressively lessen over time.

Medication for Post-traumatic Headaches

Medication is the cornerstone of treatment, as it is consistently the most effective therapeutic modality. We have available both abortive and/or preventive medication. In the first three weeks of the headaches, we usually only utilize abortive medication. If the headaches persist beyond this point, and remain moderate or severe, preventive medicine should be instituted.

Abortive Therapy

The choice of abortive therapy depends upon the type of headache that is being treated. The principle medications for treating post-traumatic tension-type headaches are the same as those outlined in Chapter 6. I often utilize the anti-inflammatories in the post-traumatic situation, so as to aid the accompanying cervical or back pain. Muscle relaxants are more helpful than in routine tension headaches, because of cervical muscle spasm. We do not want to use addicting medication on a daily basis for more than 1 or 2 weeks. If patients require excessive amounts of abortive medication, we need to consider the use of preventive medication. We do not want to create the rebound headache situation.

Typical anti-inflammatories include aspirin, ibuprofen, and naproxen. Muscle relaxants such as Flexeril or Robaxin are often helpful, but fatigue is always a problem with this class of medication. For a complete discussion of abortive medications, see Chapters 2 and 6.

Abortive therapy for post-traumatic migraine headaches follows the same guidelines as for routine migraine headaches, as outlined in Chapter 2. Antiemetic medications are helpful for many patients. The primary migraine abortives are as follows: Extra Strength Excedrin, Aspirin Free Excedrin, naproxen (Naprosyn or Anaprox), ibuprofen (Motrin), ketorolac (Toradol), Midrin, Norgesic Forte, butalbital compounds (such as fiorinal, Fioricet, Esgic, Fiorinal with codeine, and Phrenilin), ergots (such as cafergot pills or suppositories and Ergostat sublingual tablets), DHE injections or nasal spray, sumatriptan injections, corticosteroids, narcotics, and sedatives. For a discussion of these, see Chapter 2.

Most patients with migraine, and the majority of patients with post-traumatic migraine, simply require abortive medications for their headaches. However, if the migraines are frequent and/or severe, we need to progress to daily preventive therapy. The decision as to when to progress to daily preventive therapy is a difficult one, but most patients with severe post-traumatic migraines also suffer from daily headaches, and they usually benefit from preventive medication.

Preventive Medication for Post-traumatic Headaches

During the first 2 to 3 weeks of the post-trauma period, abortive medications such as anti-inflammatories are usually employed. Most patients do not need daily preventive medication, and the post-traumatic headaches decrease steadily over time. However, after the initial period, if the migraine-type headaches remain frequent (at least one or two per week) or the CDH is moderate or severe, patients may benefit from prophylactic medication.

The most commonly employed preventives for the post-traumatic headaches are the antidepressants, particularly amitriptyline (Elavil) or nortriptyline (Pamelor), and the beta blockers. The anti-inflammatories often serve a dual purpose, functioning as both abortives and preventives. The antidepressants that are sedating, particularly amitriptyline, often decrease the daily headaches, migraines, and the associated insomnia. In severe cases, we need to use both a beta blocker and an antidepressant. The selection of preventive medication differs depending upon whether there is associated insomnia, GI problems, etc., and which headache type is predominant. Chapters 3 and 7 discuss antidepressants and beta blockers for migraine and tension headache.

Although the first choices for prevention medication in the post-traumatic situation are usually antidepressants and/or beta blockers, alternative medications may be utilized. Calcium blockers (verapamil) are used for migraines as a first line therapy. Valproate (Depakote), methysergide (Sansert), and MAO inhibitors (phenelzine) are employed if initial approaches have not been successful. IV DHE, used repetitively in the office or in the hospital, is very useful with severe post-traumatic headaches. I use IV DHE relatively early in the patient's course, often after 1 or 2 months, if the headaches are very severe. Concurrently, daily preventive medication is employed in these patients. See Chapters 3 and 7 for discussions of preventive medication.

Occipital Nerve Injections for Neuralgia and Unilateral Headache Syndromes

Many patients with migraine (almost 20%) suffer intermittently from occipital neuralgia. Tenderness about the occipital nerve area is seen in many different headache syndromes. Injections in the occipital area with corticosteroids and/or lidocaine are often helpful for these patients. In addition to benefitting occipital neuralgia, occipital nerve blockade is helpful for cluster headache and cluster variants, such as chronic paroxysmal hemicrania.

Occipital Neuralgia

The first several segments of the spinal cord are important in generating posterior occipital pain, with the dorsal ramus of C2 continuing on to the scalp as the occipital nerve. Occipital neuralgia is usually sharp, ice-pick, or lancinating pain. The pain may be severe, and at times is referred to the periorbital area. Tenderness about the occipital nerve is usually elicited with palpation. Hypesthesia is present in the greater occipital nerve dermatome. The occipital nerve may be injured with trauma (as in the whiplash type of injury), it may be involved in herpes zoster

TABLE 13.2. Characteristics of Occipital Neuralgia.

Common in migraineurs (almost $\frac{1}{3}$ of migraineurs experience occipital neuralgia)
Trauma is frequently a cause
The pain is often burning, or may be stabbing or lancinating
Hypesthesia is found in the greater occipital nerve dermatome
Cortisone and/or marcaine blocks are often helpful
NSAIDs, antidepressants, and carbamazepine may decrease the pain

(shingles), in cervical pathology, or it may simply be irritated in migraineurs through unknown mechanisms. Although medications such as antidepressants, anti-inflammatories, or carbamazepine (Tegretol) may be needed, many patients with occipital neuralgia respond to injections. (See Table 13.2)

Injection Technique for Greater Occipital Nerve Block

The same technique is used whether we are treating occipital neuralgia, cluster headache, or posterior occipital pain.

There is one greater and one lesser occipital nerve on each side. I occasionally block the lesser occipital nerve that pierces the sternocleidomastoid below the ear. The greater occipital nerve is involved in pain much more frequently than the lesser occipital nerve. Many patients are tender over the nerve, and injecting at the point of tenderness is effective. The nerve runs along the half-way point between the occipital protuberance and the superior nuchal line. Palpating for the arterial pulse may be helpful.

Swab the area with alcohol, and ask the patient where tenderness is maximal; this is usually a good place to inject. However, with certain conditions, such as cluster headache, there often is no tenderness. Using a 25 gauge syringe with a $\frac{5}{8}$ inch needle, I usually mix 2% lidocaine, 1 or 1.5 cc, with betamethasone, 4 or 6 mg. Alternatively, Depo-Medrol may be used, from 40 to 80 mg. Marcaine, 0.25%, may be used as the anesthetic. I usually inject both the anesthetic and steroid, but at times one or the other may be just as effective. Some patients do better with the anesthetic, and others with the cortisone. The advantage of using only an anesthetic agent for nerve blocks or trigger point injections is that repeated injections may be performed, whereas steroid injections need to be limited. However, the steroid usually provides longer term relief.

The short needle helps to insure that we will not be entering the subarachnoid space. Feeling the bony resistance of the occipital bone also aids in telling us that we are not in the subarachnoid space. I inject $\frac{1}{2}$ cc at this point, and then withdraw the needle to just below the skin; $\frac{1}{2}$ cc is then injected medially and $\frac{1}{2}$ cc laterally, about the tender area over the occipital nerve. The area is then massaged for 1 or 2 minutes. Side effects from occipital area injections are rare, and primarily involve the very unlikely possibility of infection. "Dimpling" or discoloration of the skin may occur with corticosteroids, and that is the reason why I limit steroid injections. If patients require repeated injections, I usually use pure lidocaine or Marcaine, without cortisone. All injections in the occipital area should be limited, however, to prevent repeated trauma to the occipital nerve.

Chronic Paroxysmal Hemicrania (CPH) Continua

CPH is a variation on chronic cluster headache. Since CPH is rare, a work-up, including an MRI, is usually indicated. It is necessary to exclude a tumor (particularly pituitary) or an aneurysm. CPH is seen primarily (but not exclusively) in young women, with the typical onset from age 25 to 35. The maximal pain is usually about the eye, temple, and forehead, and, to a lesser degree, in the occiput or periaural areas. The pain is usually unilateral. Five to 20 attacks of pain occur each day, lasting from several minutes to (rarely) as long as 50 minutes. The attack typically lasts between 10 and 15 minutes. The severe pain may awaken patients from sleep, and there is no increase at one particular time of the day. Eye tearing, nasal stuffiness or rhinorrhea, conjunctival injection, and Horner's syndrome may occur. In some patients, head movement or flexion may precipitate the attack of pain. The pain is usually severe and debilitating, as it is with cluster headache.

Medication Treatment of CPH

CPH is almost always relieved by indomethacin (Indocin). If indomethacin does not help, the diagnosis of CPH is in doubt.

The dose of indomethacin varies greatly, with some patients requiring as little as 25 mg per day and others needing 250 mg or more. Although the Indocin SR 75 mg renders dosing more convenient, the 25 or 50 mg capsules, taken throughout the day, may be more effective. Patients may titrate their own dose, for at times the attacks may decrease in severity. Usually, when Indocin is tapered or stopped, the attacks resume, but long term remissions may occur. Indomethacin should be taken with food, as GI upset is very common. Although headache may occur as a side effect of indomethacin, it is not common in patients with preexisting headaches. Cognitive side effects, such as fatigue, lightheadedness, and mood swings, may be a problem with indomethacin. Retinal or corneal problems have been reported with long term use of indomethacin. As with all of the anti-inflammatories, renal and hepatic functions need to be monitored through blood tests.

Corticosteroids, naproxen, and calcium blockers (verapamil) may provide some benefit, but these have limited usefulness in CPH. Fluoxetine (Prozac) may be of benefit in some patients.

TABLE 13.3. Clinical Characteristics of Hemicrania Continua.

Unilateral severe pain lasting 5–60 minutes, usually pulsating or throbbing
Nausea or photophobia may be present with the severe pain
Attacks occur 3–5 times per 24 hours
Underlying unilateral aching, dull pain
Patients may be awakened from sleep with the severe pain
Icepick stabbing pain throughout the day
Physical exertion increases the pain in many patients
Alcohol may increase the pain.
Indomethacin is effective in $\frac{4}{5}$ of patients.
Ergots, NSAIDs, tricyclics, or verapamil are effective for some patients

Hemicrania Continua

Hemicrania continua occurs in men and women at all ages. These patients have unilateral dull pain, with icepick pains intermittently during the day, and focal, intense pain lasting minutes. The pain is often increased with alcohol or physical exertion. Typical migrainous features may be present, such as sensitivity to light and accompanying nausea. There are many patients who do not fulfill all of these criteria, but who have unilateral dull or throbbing pain on a daily basis, with migraine features. They usually also experience intermittent icepick-type jabbing pains.

Indomethacin, as outlined in the above section on CPH, is the drug of choice with hemicrania continua. Patients who fit some but not all of the criteria for hemicrania continua also may respond to indomethacin. If indomethacin is not able to be used, or is not helpful, then proceeding along migraine prevention lines is required. Amitriptyline, naproxen, and calcium blockers may be helpful. (See Table 13.3)

Exertional and Sexual Headaches

Exertional headaches are frequently found in both migraine sufferers and nonheadache patients. Although organic pathology needs to be excluded, it has become apparent that, in the vast majority of people, these headaches are benign.

Exertional headaches are more common in patients over the age of 40, occurring with the same frequency in both women and men. The headache occurs after exercise (such as weight lifting, aerobics, jogging, or sexual intercourse), and may be brief in duration, 15 to 20 minutes, or prolonged, lasting up to 1 day. In patients with coexisting migraine or cluster headaches, the exertional headache is usually of the same type.

Although any activity that increases intracranial pressure may produce an exertional headache, certain exercises are more likely to lead to a headache. These include weight lifting, "heading" the ball in soccer, jogging, diving, and sexual activity. The lower impact activities, such as walking, swimming, treadmilling, and biking, will not usually produce exercise-induced headaches. Patients who have recently begun physical fitness programs are more likely to experience exertional migraines.

Any neurologic problem that becomes apparent with increasing intracranial pressure may manifest itself during sexual activity. Meningitis, subarachnoid hemorrhage, and stroke may become apparent during sex. Occasionally, headaches occurring during sexual activity originate from problems outside of the CNS, such as an obstructive lesion of the lower aorta. However, sex-induced headaches are generally benign, without intracranial or other pathology. Although the term "coital cephalgia" was coined in the 1960s, other activities, such as masturbation or simply assuming the position for intercourse, may produce a headache.

The sexual headache varies in length from minutes to hours, and the severity may be mild or, more frequently, moderate to severe. The two primary pathophysiologic mechanisms involve vascular components and muscle contraction. One other pathophysiologic mechanism is the headache with low CSF pressure, noted in a few patients with sexual headaches.

The timing of the headaches is variable, but they usually occur just prior to orgasm. The headache with sexual intercourse is usually occipital, but it may be generalized. Stopping intercourse when the headache begins may lessen the length or duration of the headache. It has recently been reported that sex will occasionally stop a migraine headache in progress, and this has been seen in several cluster headache patients as well.

Workup of Exertional and Sexual Headaches

Subarachnoid hemorrhage from aneurysm or AVM, and tumors that block the ventricular outflow, such as a colloid cyst of the third ventricle, need to be excluded. Other organic pathologies to be considered include tumors of the posterior fossa, chronic subdural hematomas, basilar impression, platybasia, Arnold–Chiari, and the very rare cases of pheochromocytoma, hypoglycemia, hypertension, hyperthyroidism, COPD, meningitis, or stroke.

In the acute situation, CAT scan and lumbar puncture are important in ruling out subarachnoid hemorrhage. Although MRI is not as useful in the acute situation with the possibility of bleeding, it is extremely useful in looking for other possibilities, including tumors. For most patients, the workup of exertional headache includes checking blood pressure, drawing a routine thyroid screen, and, most importantly, doing a CAT scan with infusion or an MRI of the brain. In the acute situation where subarachnoid hemorrhage is suspected, lumbar puncture may be necessary if the CAT scan is negative. MR Angiography (MRA) is a good non-invasive screening test for aneurysms.

Treatment of Exertional Headaches

If possible, avoiding the precipitating exercise may be useful, but for patients not willing or able to do this, two primary treatments may be used: anti-inflammatories and propranolol.

The anti-inflammatories indomethacin (Indocin) and naproxen (Naprosyn, Anaprox) have been the most commonly used medications. Ibuprofen (Motrin) or flurbiprofen (Ansaid) are also effective for some patients. The anti-inflammatory is usually given $\frac{1}{2}$ to 2 hours prior to the activity. The effective dose varies widely, but the usual dosages are as follows: indomethacin, 50 to 75 mg; Naprosyn, 500 mg, or Anaprox D.S., one tablet (550 mg); ibuprofen, 600 to 800 mg; flurbiprofen (Ansaid), one or two of the 100 mg tablets.

Propranolol (Inderal) has also been utilized at a dose of 20 to 60 mg given $\frac{1}{2}$ or 1 hour prior to the exercise. Fatigue and decreased exercise tolerance are always potential problems with propranolol.

Abortive treatment of the headache follows the usual therapy for tension or migraine headaches. Therapy consists of the application of ice to the head, lying down in a dark room, and taking medication. For a discussion of the abortive treatment of migraine and tension headache, please see Chapters 2 and 6.

Lumbar Puncture Headache

Headache after a lumbar puncture (LP) is a major problem, occurring in 30% to 35% of patients. Post-LP headache may occur in any person, but women with a previous history of headache seem particularly prone to developing this problem. Younger patients, particularly those with lower body mass, are more susceptible. The position of the patient after the LP, experience of the person performing the procedure, and amount of CSF taken during the LP do not appear to increase the risk of developing the headache. Psychological factors play a lesser role than was once thought. Smaller LP needles are an important factor in avoiding the headache. New LP needles have been developed that may decrease the incidence of post LP headache.

The headache will usually be present within several days, but a delay may occur of up to 2 weeks. The pain may be frontal, occipital, or in the cervical and shoulder regions. The headache is positional in nature, with increased pain sitting or standing, and relief with the supine position. The pain may be throbbing, pounding, or simply a severe ache.

Patients may report symptoms typical for migraine, such as nausea, visual symptoms, photophobia, dizziness, and vertigo. In addition, cervical pain and spasm are often present, with nuchal rigidity. This may confuse the situation, as meningitis becomes a consideration. Meningitis following LP is exceedingly rare, usually presenting a problem only in immunocompromised patients with sepsis. (See Table 13.4)

TABLE 13.4. Features of Lumbar Puncture Headache.

Headache is more common in younger women with lower body mass
Headache is greatly increased sitting, decreased supine
Shaking the head increases the pain
Onset is usually within 48 hours
Nausea is common
Pain is aching but may be pulsating
Location may be frontal, occipital, or both
Visual blurring may occur, as may photophobia
Low back pain may be present
IV or IM caffeine is beneficial
Epidural blood patch is highly effective
Standard analgesics are only mildly effective

LP headache is almost always self limited, resolving in days to weeks. Chronic headache may persist for months or, rarely, years. The mechanism of the headache is questionable. Leakage through the dura is certainly an obvious answer, but vascular or serotonergic factors may be important as well.

Treatment of Lumbar Puncture Headache

With most patients, the headaches do resolve quickly, within days, and simple analgesics are all that are necessary. Oral caffeine may help, but usually patients cannot consume enough orally to significantly decrease the headache.

When the headache persists for more than 2 days, caffeine sodium benzoate may be given intravenously or intramuscularly. The IV caffeine is more likely to produce lasting relief. One dose of IV 500 mg caffeine is given, and this may be repeated, if necessary, in 6 hours. Caffeine and sodium benzoate is available in 2 ml amps of 250 mg caffeine per ml. This may be given IM, 250 mg every 3 to 6 hours, as needed. Patients may learn to do this at home for a number of days. With these large doses of caffeine, CNS side effects may occur, as well as tachycardia. Along with caffeine, analgesics provide a small amount of relief. Hydration is helpful to a small extent, and patients are encouraged to drink at least six glasses of liquid per day.

If the headache is severe and not improving, an epidural blood patch should be given. This is usually done several days to 1 week after the LP. Epidural injections of the patient's blood at the site of the LP are extremely effective in terminating the headache. The blood does track up and down the spinal area, thus helping the headache even if the blood is injected above or below the involved site. Twelve cc of blood are usually utilized. Pain at the injection site or radicular pain may occur with the blood patch, but rarely do these complications last more than days to weeks. Occasionally, there is a need for a second blood patch, or even a third. If the epidural blood patches fail to alleviate the symptoms, the patient is treated with standard headache prevention medications. In addition, epidural saline may be injected. This will occasionally help even when the blood patch has failed.

Appendix A

References

Migraine Headache

Anthony M, Lance JW. Monoamine oxidase inhibition in the treatment of migraine. Arch Neurol. 21:263–268; 1969.

Bockstrom T, Hammarbock S. Premenstrual syndrome—psychiatric or gynecological disorder? Headache Quarterly, Cur Tx & Res. 3(2):220; 1992.

Belgrade M, Ling L, Schleevogt M, Ettinger M, Ruiz E. Comparison of single dose meperidine, butorphanol, and dihydroergotamine in the treatment of vascular headache. Neurology. 39:590–592; 1989.

Bell R, Montoya D, Shuaib A, Lee M. A comparative trial of three agents in the treatment of acute migraine headache. Ann Emerg Med. 19:1079–1082; 1990.

Blackwell B, Marley E, Price J, Taylor D. Hypertensive interactions between monoamine oxidase inhibitors and foodstuffs. Br J Psych. 113:349–365; 1967.

Breslau N, David GD. Migraine, major depression and panic disorder: a prospective epidemiologic study of young adults. Cephalalgia. 12:85–90; 1992.

Brewerton TD, George MS. A study of the seasonal variation of migraine. Headache Quarterly, Cur Tx & Res. 2(1):55; 1991.

Brewerton TD, George MS. A study of the seasonal variation of migraine. Headache. 30:511–513; 1990.

Callaham M, Raskin N. A controlled study of dihydroergotamine in the treatment of acute migraine headache. Headache. 26:168–171; 1986.

Calton GJ, Burnett JW. Danazol and migraine. N Engl J Med. 310:721–722; 1984.

Celentano DD, Stewart WF, Lipton RB, Reed ML. Medication use and disability among migraineurs: a national probability sample survey. Headache. 32:223–228; 1992.

Couch JR, Hassanein RS. Amitriptyline in migraine prophylaxis. Arch Neurol. 36:695–699; 1979.

Couch JR, Ziegler DK, Hassanein RS. Amitriptyline in the prophylaxis of migraine. Neurology. 26:121–127; 1976.

Couch JR. Placebo effect and clinical trials in migraine therapy. Neuroepidemiology. 6:178–185; 1987.

Couturier EGM, Hering R, Steiner TJ. Weekend attacks in migraine patients: caused by caffeine withdrawal? Cephalalgia. 12:99–100; 1992.

Cruickshank JM, Neil-Dwyer G. Beta-blocker brain concentrations in man. Eur J Clin Pharmacol. 28(Suppl):21–23; 1985.

Curran DA, Hinterberger H, Lance JW. Methysergide. Rs Clin Stud Headache. 1:74–122; 1967.

Dennerstein L, Laby B, Burrows GD, Hyman GJ. Headache and sex hormone therapy. Headache. 18:146–153; 1978.

Diamond ML. Emergency department treatment of the headache patient. Headache Quarterly, Cur Tx & Res. 3(Suppl 1):28–33; 1992.

Diamond S. Treatment of migraine with isometheptene, acetaminophen, and dichloralphenazone combination: a double-blind, crossover trial. Headache. 15:282–287; 1976.

Diamond S. Menstrual migraine and non-steroidal anti-inflammatory agents. Headache. 24:52; 1984.

Diamond S, Kudrow L, Stevens J, Shapiro DB. Long-term study of propranolol in the treatment of migraine. Headache. 22:268–271; 1982.

Diamond S, Solomon GD, Freitag FG, Mehta N. Fenoprofen in the prophylaxis of migraine: a double-blind, placebo controlled study. Headache. 27:246–249; 1987.

Diamond S, Solomon GD. Pharmacologic treatment of migraine. Rat Drug Ther. 22:1–5; 1988.

Diamond S, Solomon GD, Freitag FG, Mehta ND. Long-acting propranolol in the prophylaxis of migraine. Headache. 27:70–72; 1987.

Dimsdale JE, Newton RP. Cognitive effects of beta blockers. Headache Quarterly, Cur Tx & Res. 3(3):347; 1992.

Drummond PD. Effectiveness of methysergide in relation to clinical features of migraine. Headache. 25:145–146; 1985.

Facchinetti F, Sances G, Borella P, Genazzani AR, Nappi G. Magnesium prophylaxis of menstrual migraine: effects on intracellular magnesium. Headache. 31:298–301; 1991.

Fuller GN, Guiloff RJ. Propranolol in acute migraine: a controlled study. Cephalalgia. 10:229–233; 1990.

Gallagher RM. Emergency treatment of intractable migraine. Headache. 26:74–75; 1986.

Gilbert RM, Marshman JA, Schweider M, Berg R. Caffeine content of beverages as consumed. Can Med Assoc J. 114:205–208; 1976.

Goadsby PJ, Zagami AS, Donnan GA, et al. Oral sumatriptan in acute migraine. Headache Quarterly, Cur Tx & Res. 3(2):212; 1992.

Goldstein J. Ergot pharmacology and alternative delivery systems for ergotamine derivatives. Headache Quarterly, Cur Tx Res. 3(3):345; 1992.

Gomersall JD, Stuart A. Amitriptyline in migraine prophylaxis. J Neurol Neurosurg Psych. 36:684–690; 1973.

Graham J. Cardiac and pulmonary fibrosis during methysergide therapy for headache. Am J Med Sci. 254:1–12; 1967.

Greenberg DA. Calcium channel antagonists and the treatment of migraine. Clin Neuropharmacol. 9:311–328; 1986.

Greenberg DA. Calcium channel and calcium channel antagonists. Ann Neurol. 21:317–330; 1987.

Grotemeyer K-H, Scharafinski H-W, Husstedt IW. Acetylsalicylic acid vs. metoprolol in migraine prophylaxis—a double-blind cross-over study. Headache. 30:639–641; 1990.

Hakkarainen H, Allonen H. Ergotamine vs. metoclopramide vs. their combination in acute migraine attacks. Headache. 22:10–12; 1982.

Hakkarainen H, Vapaatolo H, Gothoni G. Tolfenamic acid is as effective as ergotamine during migraine attacks. Lancet. 2:326–327; 1979.

Harden RN, Carter TD, Gilman CS. Ketorolac in acute headache management. Headache. 31:463–464; 1991.

Hauck AJ, Edwards WD, Danielson GK, Mullany CJ, Bresnahan DR. Mitral and aortic valve disease associated with ergotamine therapy for migraine. Headache Quarterly, Cur Tx & Res. 2(1):58; 1991.

Hering R, Kuritzky A. Sodium valproate in the prophylactic treatment of migraine: a double-blind study versus placebo. Cephalalgia. 12:81–84; 1992.

Hokkanen E, Waltimo O, Kallanranta T. Toxic effects of ergotamine used for migraine. Headache. 18:95–98; 1978.

Holroyd KA, Penzien DB, Cordingley GE. Propranolol in the management of recurrent migraine: a meta-analytic review. Headache. 31:333–340; 1991.

Holroyd KA, Penzien DB. Pharmacological versus non-pharmacological prophylaxis of recurrent migraine headache: A meta-analytic review of clinical trials. Headache Quarterly, Cur Tx & Res. 2(1):59; 1991.

Johnson ES, Ratcliffe DM, Wilkinson M. Naproxen sodium in the treatment of migraine. Cephalalgia. 5:5–10; 1985.

Jones J, Sklar D, Dougherty J, White W. Randomized double-blind trial of IV prochlorperazine for the treatment of acute headache. JAMA. 261:1174–1176; 1989.

Jonsdottir M, Meyer JS, Rogers RL. Efficacy, side effects and tolerance compared during headache treatment with three different calcium blockers. Headache. 27:364–369; 1987.

Joseph R, Steiner T, Schultz L, Rose CF. Platelet activity and selective beta-blockage in migraine prophylaxis: a case for preferring beta1 adrenoceptor blockers. Stroke. 19:704–708; 1988.

Klapper JA, Stanton J. Clinical experience with patient administered subcutaneous dihydroergotamine mesylate in refractory headaches. Headache Quarterly, Cur Tx & Res. 3(3):345; 1992.

Klapper JA. Emergency management of benign headaches. Headache Quarterly, Cur Tx & Res. 3(2):160–163; 1992.

Klapper J, Stanton J. A comparison of dihydroergotamine, dexamethasone and placebo in the treatment of acute migraine headache. Cephalalgia. 11(Suppl 11):159–161; 1991a.

Kloster R, Nestvold K, Vilming ST. A double-blind study of ibuprofen versus placebo in the treatment of acute migraine attacks. Cephalalgia. 12:169–171; 1992.

Koella WP. CNS-related side effects of beta-blockers with special reference to mechanisms of action. Eur J Clin Pharmacol. 28:55–63; 1985.

Krause KH, Bleicher MA. DHE nasal spray in the treatment of migraine attacks. Cephalagia. 5(Suppl 3):138–139; 1985.

Kudrow L. The relationship of headache frequency to hormonal use in migraine. Headache. 15:36–40; 1975.

Lader M. Combined use of tricyclic antidepressants and monoamine oxidase inhibitors. J Clin Psychiatry. 44:20–24; 1983.

Lance JW. The pharmacotherapy of migraine. Med J Aust. 144:85–88; 1986.

Laska EM, Sunshine A, Mueller F, et al. Caffeine as an analgesic adjuvant. JAMA. 251:1711–1718; 1984.

Lichten EM, Bennett RS, Whitty AJ, Daoud Y. Efficacy of danazol in the control of hormonal migraine. Headache Quarterly, Cur Tx & Res. 3(2):219; 1992.

Lindegaard KF, Ovrelid L, Sjaastad O. Naproxen in the prevention of migraine attacks. A double-blind placebo-controlled crossover study. Headache. 20:96–98; 1980.

Magos AL, Zilkha KJ, Studd JWW. Treatment of menstrual migrine by oestradiol implants. J Neurol Neurosurg Psych. 46:1044–1046; 1983.

Markley HG, Cheronis JCD, Piepho RW. Verapamil in prophylactic therapy of migraine. Neurology. 34:963–976; 1984.

Massiou H, Serrurier D, Lasserre O, Bousser M-G. Effectiveness of oral diclofenac in the acute treatment of common migraine attacks: a double-blind study versus placebo. Cephalalgia. 11:59–63; 1991.

Mathew NT. Prophylaxis of migraine and mixed headache: a randomized controlled study. Headache. 21:105–109; 1981.

Mathew NT, Reuveni U, Perez F. Transformed or evolutive migraine. Headache. 27:102–106; 1987.

McEwen J, O'Connor H, Dinsdale H. Treatment of migraine with intramuscular chlorpromazine. Ann Emerg Med. 16:758–763; 1987.

Medina JL, Diamond S. The role of diet in migraine. Headache. 18:31–34; 1978.

Meyer JS. Calcium channel blockers in the prophylactic treatment of vascular headache. Ann Intern Med. 102:395–397; 1985.

Meyer JS, Dowell R, Mathew N, Hardenburg J. Clinical and hemodynamic treatment of vascular headaches with verapamil. Headache. 24:313–321; 1984.

Mitchelson F. Pharmacological agents affecting emesis, a review (Part I). Headache Quarterly, Cur Tx & Res. 3(3):347; 1992.

Mondell BE. Office management of acute headache. Headache Quarterly, Cur Tx & Res. 3(Suppl 1):4–9; 1992.

Monro J, Brostoff J, Carini C, Zilkha K. Food allergy in migraine: study of food allergy and RAST. Lancet. 2:1; 1980.

Nestvold K. Naproxen and naproxen sodium in acute migraine. Cephalalgia. 6(Suppl 4):81–84; 1986.

Neuman M, Demarez JP, Harmey JL, Le Bastard B, Cauquil J. Prevention of migraine attacks through the use of dihydroergotamine. Int J Clin Pharmacol Res. 6:11–13; 1986.

Olerud B, Gustavsson C-L, Furberg B. Nadolol and propranolol in migraine management. Headache. 26:490–493; 1986.

Olesen J. Role of calcium entry blockers in the prophylaxis of migraine. Eur Neurol. 25(Suppl 1):72–79; 1986b.

Orlando RC, Moyer P, Barnett TB. Methysergide therapy and constrictive pericarditis. Ann Intern Med. 88:213–214; 1978.

Pearce I, Frank GJ, Pearce JMS. Ibuprofen compared with paracetamol in migraine. Practitioner. 227:465–467; 1983.

Peatfield R. Drugs and the treatment of migraine. Trends Pharmacol Sci. 9:141–145; 1988.

Peatfield RC, Fozard JR, Rose FC. Drug treatment of migraine. In: Handbook of Clinical Neurology, Vol. 48. FC Rose, ed. Amsterdam; Elsevier Science Publishing: 173–216; 1986.

Peroutka S. Sumatriptan in acute migraine: pharmacology and review of world experience. Headache. 30(Suppl 2):554–560; 1990.

Peroutka S, Allen GS. The calcium antagonist properties of cyproheptadine: implications for antimigraine action. Neurology. 34:304–309; 1984.

Peroutka SJ, Banghart SB, Allen GS. Relative potency and selectivity of calcium channel antagonists used in the treatment of migraine. Headache. 24:55–58; 1984.

Peters BH, Fraim CJ, Masel BE. Comparison of 650 mg aspirin and 1,000 mg acetaminophen with each other, and with placebo in moderately severe headache. Am J Med. (Suppl June 14):36–42; 1983.

Powles TJ. Prevention of migrainous headache by tamoxifen. Lancet. 2:1344; 1986.

Pradalier A, Rancurel G, Dordain G, et al. Acute migraine attack therapy—comparison of naproxen sodium and an ergotamine tartrate compound. Cephalalgia. 5:107–113; 1985.

Primavera III JP, Kaiser RS. Non-pharmacological treatment of headache: is less more? Headache. 32:393–395; 1992.

Rapaport A, Weeks R, Sheftell F, et al. Analgesic rebound headache: theoretical and practical implications. Cephalalgia. 5(Suppl 3):448–449; 1985.

Rapoport AM. The diagnosis of migraine and tension-type headache, then and now. Headache Quarterly, Cur Tx & Res. 3(3):348; 1992.

Rapoport AM, Silberstein SD. Emergency treatment of headache. Headache Quarterly, Cur Tx & Res. 3(3):346; 1992.

Raskin NH. Repetitive intravenous dihydroergotamine as therapy for intractable migraine. Neurology. 36:995–997; 1986.

Raskin NH. Pharmacology of migraine. Annu Rev Pharmacol Toxicol. 21:463–478; 1981.

Raskin N. Treatment of status migranosus: the American experience. Headache. 30(Suppl 2):550–553; 1990.

Raskin NH, Schwartz RK. Interval therapy of migraine; long-term results. Headache. 20:336–340; 1980.

Riopleel RJ, McCans JL. A pilot study of the calcium antagonist diltiazem in migraine syndrome prophylaxis. Can J Neurol Sci. 9:269; 1982.

Robbins L, Remmes A. Outpatient Repetitive Intravenous Dihydroergotamine. Headache. 32, No. 9:455–458; 1992.

Rosen JA. Observations on the efficacy of propranolol for the prophylaxis of migraine. Ann Neurol. 13:92–93; 1983.

Ross-Lee L, Headlewood V, Tyrer JH, Eadie MJ. Aspirin treatment of migraine attacks: plasma drug level data. Cephalalgia. 2:9–14; 1982b.

Ryan Sr. RE Comparative study of nadolol and propranolol in prophylactic treatment of migraine. Am Heart J. 108:1156–1158; 1984.

Saadah HA. Abortive headache therapy with intramuscular dihydroergotamine. Headache Quarterly, Cur Tx & Res. 3(3):345; 1992.

Saadah HA. Abortive headache therapy in the office with intravenous dihydroergotamine plus prochlorperazine. Headache Quarterly, Cur Tx & Res. 3(3):345; 1992.

Saadah HA. Abortive headache therapy in the office with intravenous dihydroergotamine plus prochlorperazine. Headache. 32:143–146; 1992.

Sances G, Martignoni E, Fioroni L, Blandini F, Facchinetti F, Nappi G. Naproxen sodium in menstrual migraine prophylaxis: a double-blind placebo controlled study. Headache. 30:705–709; 1990.

Sargent J, Solbach P, Coyne L, et al. Results of a controlled, experimental outcome study of nondrug treatments for the control of migraine headaches. J Behav Med. 9:291–323; 1986.

Sargent JD, Baumel B, Peters K, et al. Aborting a migraine attack: naproxen sodium vs ergotamine plus caffeine. Headache. 28:263–266; 1988.

Schiffman S, Buckley CE, Sampson HA, et al. Aspartame and susceptibility to headache. N Engl J Med. 317:1181–1185; 1987.

Schulman EA, Silberstein SD. Symptomatic and prophylactic treatment of migraine and tension-type headache. Neurology. 42(Suppl 2):16–21; 1992.

Scopp AL. MSG and hydrolyzed vegetable protein induced headache: review and case studies. Headache. 31:107–110; 1991.

Selby G, Lance JW. Observations on 500 cases of migraine and allied vascular headache. J Neurol Neurosurg Psychiatry. 23:23–32; 1960.

Silberstein SD. Appropriate use of abortive medication in headache treatment. Headache Quarterly, Cur Tx & Res. 3(2):212; 1992.

Silberstein SD. The role of sex hormones in headache. Headache Quarterly, Cur Tx & Res. 3(3):349; 1992.

Silberstein SD. Advances in understanding the pathophysiology of headache. Neurology. 42(Suppl 2):6–10; 1992.

Silberstein SD. The role of sex hormones in headache. Neurology. 42(Suppl 2):37–42; 1992.

Silberstein SD. Evaluation and emergency treatment of headache. Headache. 32:396–407; 1992.

Silberstein SD, Schulman EA, Hopkins MM. Repetitive intravenous DHE in the treatment of refractory headache. Headache. 30:334–339, 1990.

Solomon GD. Management of the headache patient with medical illness. Clin J Pain. 5:95–99; 1989.

Solomon GD, Griffith Steel MD, Spaccavento LJ. Verapamil prophylaxis of migraine. JAMA. 250:2500–2502; 1983.

Sommerville BW. Estrogen withdrawal migraine. 1. Duration of exposure and attempted prophylaxis by premenstrual estrogen administration. Neurology. 25:239–244; 1975.

Spiegel K, Kalb R, Pasternak GW. Analgesic activity of tricyclic antidepressants. Ann Neurol. 13:462–465; 1983.

Steiner TJ, Joseph R. Practical experience of beta-blockage in migraine: a personal view. Postgrad Med J. 60(Suppl 2):56–60; 1984.

Stensrud P, Sjaastad O. Clinical trial of a new antibradykinin, anti-inflammatory drug, ketoprofen, in migraine prophylaxis. Headache. 14:96–100; 1974.

Stone AB, Pearlstein TB, Brown WA. Fluoxetine in the treatment of late luteal phase dysphoric disorder. Headache Quarterly, Cur Tx & Res. 3(2):219; 1992.

Subcutaneous Sumatriptan International Study Group. Treatment of migraine attacks with sumatriptan. N Engl J Med. 325:316–321; 1991.

Tek D, McClellan D, Olshaker M, Allen C, Arthur D. A prospective, double-blind study of metoclopramide hydrochloride for the control of migraine in the emergency department. Ann Emerg Med. 19:1083–1087; 1990.

Tfelt-Hansen P. Efficacy of Beta-blockers in migraine. Cephalalgia. 6(Suppl 5): 15–24; 1986.

Tfelt-Hansen P, Olesen J, Aebelholt-Krabbe A, et al. A double-blind study of metoclopramide in the treatment of migraine attacks. J Neurol Neurosurg Psychiat. 43:369–371; 1980.

Tfelt-Hansen P, Paalzow L, Ibraheem JJ. Bioavailability of sublingual ergotamine. Br J Clin Pharmacol. 13:239–240; 1982b.

Treves TA, Streiffler M, Korczyn AD. Naproxen sodium versus ergotamine tartrate in the treatment of acute migraine attacks. Headache. 32:280–282; 1992.

Tucker JS, Whalen RE. Premenstrual syndrome. Headache Quarterly, Cur Tx & Res. 3(3):349; 1992.

Turkewitz LJ, Casaly JS, Dawson GA, Wirth O. Phenelzine therapy for headache patients with concomitant depression and anxiety. Headache. 32:203–208; 1992.

Vincent FM. Migraine responsive to danazol. Neurology 35:618; 1985.

Wainscott G, Sullivan FM, Volans GN, Wilkinson M. The outcome of pregnancy in women suffering from migraine. Postgrad Med J. 54:98–102; 1978.

Ward TN, Scott G. Dihydroergotamine suppositories in a headache clinic. Headache. 31:465–466; 1991.

Welch KMA, Ellis DJ, Keenan PA. Successful migraine prophylaxis with naproxen sodium. Neurology. 35:1304–1310; 1985.

Wilkinson M. Treatment of acute migraine: the British experience. Headache. 30(Suppl 2):545–549; 1990.

Wood AJJ. Pharmacologic differences between beta blockers. Am Heart J. 108:1070–1076; 1984.

Yardi Y, Rabey JM, Streifler M. Migraine attacks: alleviation by an inhibitor of prostaglandin synthesis and action. Neurology. 26:447–450, 1976.

Zahavi I, Chagnac A, Hering R, et al. Prevalence of Raynaud's phenomenon in patients with migraine. Arch Intern Med. 144(4):742–744; 1984.

Ziegler DK. Headache and migraine. Headache Quarterly, Cur Tx & Res. 3(3): 340; 1992.

Ziegler DK, Ellis DJ. Naproxen in prophylaxis of migraine. Arch Neurol. 42:582–584; 1985.

Tension Headache

Barclay CL, Shuaib A, Montoya D, Seland TP, Thomas HG. Response of non-migrainous headaches to chlorpromazine. Headache. 30:85–87; 1990.

Diamond S, Baltes BJ. Chronic tension headache treated with amitriptyline—a double blind study. Headache. 11:110–116; 1971.

Glass DE. Tension headache and some psychiatric aspects of headache. Headache Quarterly, Cur Tx & Res. 3(3):262–269; 1992.

Henry P, Dartigues JF, Benetier MP. Ergotamine and analgesic induced headaches. In: Migraine: Proceedings 5th International Migraine Symposium. FC Rose, ed. London; Karger: 197–205; 1984.

Kudrow L. Muscle contraction headaches. In: Handbook of Clinical Neurology, Vol. 48. FC Rose, ed. Amsterdam; Elsevier Science Publishing: 343–352; 1986.

Kudrow L. Paradoxical effects of frequent analgesic use. Adv Neurol. 33:335–341; 1982.

Lader M. Combined use of tricyclic antidepressants and monoamine oxidase inhibitors. J Clin Psychiatry. 44:20–24; 1983.

Lance JW. Tension headache. In: Mechanism and Management of Headache, 4th edition. Butterworth; London/Boston: 100–120; 1982.

Lance JW, Curan DA. Treatment of chronic tension headache. Lancet. 1: 1236–1239; 1964.

Magni G. The use of antidepressants in the treatment of chronic pain. A review of the current evidence. Headache Quarterly, Cur Tx & Res. 3(2): 233; 1992.

Mathew NT. Prophylaxis of migraine and mixed headache. A randomized controlled study. Headache. 21:105–109; 1981.

Mathew NT, Ali S. Valproate in the treatment of persistent chronic daily headache. An open label study. Headache. 31:71–74; 1991.

Mathew NT, Reuveni U, Perez F. Transformed or evolutive migraine. Headache. 27:102–106; 1987.

Olesen J. Management of acute nonvascular headache: the Danish experience. Headache. 30(Suppl 2):541–544; 1990.

Primavera III JP, Kaiser RS. Non-pharmacological treatment of headache: is less more? Headache. 32:393–395; 1992.

Rapoport AM. The diagnosis of migraine and tension-type headache, then and now. Headache Quarterly, Cur Tx & Res. 3(3):348; 1992.

Rapaport A, Weeks R, Sheftell F. Analgesic rebound headache: theoretical and practical implications. Cephalalgia. 5(Suppl 3):448–449; 1985.

Raskin NH. Repetitive intravenous dihydroergotamine as treatment for intractable migraine. Neurology. 36:995–997; 1986.

Raskin NH, Hosobuchi Y, Lamb S. Headache may arise from perturbation of the brain. Headache. 27:416–420; 1987.

Saper JR. Changing perspectives on chronic headache. Clin J Pain. 2:19–28; 1986.

Saper JR. Drug treatment of headache: changing concepts and treatment strategies. Semin Neurol. 7:178–191; 1987.

Schulman EA, Silberstein SD. Symptomatic and prophylactic treatment of migraine and tension-type headache. Neurology. 42(Suppl 2):16–21; 1992.

Sheftell FD. Chronic daily headache. Neurology. 42(Suppl 2):32–36; 1992.

Solomon S, Lipton RB, Newman LC. Clinical features of chronic daily headache. Headache. 32:325–329; 1992.

Turkewitz LJ, Casaly JS, Dawson GA, Wirth O. Phenelzine therapy for headache patients with concomitant depression and anxiety. Headache. 32:203–208; 1992.

Ziegler DK. Tension-muscle contraction headaches. A review. In: Updating in Headache. eds. V Pfaffenrath, P-O Lundberg, O Sjaastad, Springer-Verlag; Berlin: 315–320; 1985.

Cluster Headache

Anderson P, Jespersen L. Dihydroergotamine nasal spray in the treatment of attacks of cluster headache. Cephalalgia. 6:51–54; 1986.

Anthony M. Arrest of attacks of cluster headache by local steroid injection of the occipital nerve. In: Migraine: Clinical and Research Advances. FC Rose, ed. Basel; Karger: 169; 1985.

Barre F. Cocaine as an abortive agent in cluster headache. Headache. 22:69–73; 1982.

Campbell JK. Cluster headache. In: Management of headache. FC Rose, ed. New York; Raven Press: 115–126; 1988.

Couch JR, Ziegler D. Prednisone therapy for cluster headache. Headache. 17:15–18; 1977.

Diamond S, Freitag FG, Prager J, Gandhi S. Treatment of intractable cluster. Headache. 26:42–46; 1986.

Ekbom K. Lithium for cluster headache: review of the literature and preliminary results of long-term treatments. Headache. 21:132–139; 1981.

Ekbom K, Lindgren L, Nilsson BY, Hardebo JE, Waldenlind E. Retro-gasserian glycerol injection in the treatment of chronic cluster headache. Cephalalgia. 7:21–27; 1987.

Fusco BM, Geppetti P, Fancicullacci M, Sicuteri F. Local application of capsaicin for the treatment of cluster headache and idiopathic trigeminal neuralgia. Cephalalgia. 11(Suppl 2):234–235; 1991.

Gabe IJ, Spierings ELH. Prophylactic treatment of cluster headache with verapamil. Headache. 29:167–168; 1989.

Hardebo JE. On pain mechanisms in cluster headache. Headache. 31:91–106; 1991.

Hassenbusch SJ, Kunkel RS, Kosmorsky GS, Covington EC, Pillay PK. Trigeminal cisternal injection of glycerol for treatment of chronic intractable cluster headaches. Headache Quarterly, Cur Tx & Res. 3(2):222; 1992.

Hering R, Kuritzky A. Sodium valproate in the treatment of cluster headache: an open clinical trial. Cephalalgia. 9:195–198; 1989.

Kitrelle J, Grouse D, Seybold M. Cluster headache, local anesthetic abortive agents. Arch Neurol. 41:496–498; 1985.

Kittrelle JP, Grouse DS, Seybold M. Cluster headache: local anaesthetic abortive agents. Arch Neurol. 42:406–408; 1985.

Klapper JA. Recent advances in the treatment of cluster headache. Headache Quarterly, Cur Tx & Res. 3(Suppl 1):10–15; 1992.

Kudrow L. Cluster Headache, Mechanisms and Management. Oxford: Oxford University Press; 1980.

Kudrow L. Cluster headaches. In: Migraine: Clinical, Therapeutic, Conceptual and Research Aspects. JN, Blau ed. London; Chapman & Hall: 113–133; 1987.

Kudrow L. Cluster headache. Clin J Pain. 5:29–38; 1989.

Kudrow L. Lithium prophylaxis for chronic cluster headache. Headache. 17: 15–18; 1977.

Kudrow L. Subchronic cluster headache. Headache. 27:197–200; 1987.

Kudrow L. Response of cluster headache attacks to oxygen inhalation. Headache. 21:1–4; 1981.

Kudrow L. Comparative results of prednisone, methysergide and lithium therapy in cluster headache. In: Current Concepts in Migraine Research. R Croons, ed. New York; Raven Press: 159–163; 1978.

Manzoni GC, Micieli G, Granella F, Tassorelli C, Zanferrari C, Cavallini A. Cluster headache—course over ten years in 189 patients. Grappi Award Lecture, Vth International Headache Congress, Washington DC: 1991.

Mather PJ, Silberstein SD, Schulman EA, Hopkins MM. The treatment of cluster headache with repetitive intravenous dihydroergotamine. Headache Quarterly, Cur Tx & Res. 3(2):222; 1992.

Mathew N. Clinical subtypes of cluster headache and response to lithium therapy. Headache. 18:26–80; 1978.

Mathew NT. Cluster headache. Neurology. 42(Suppl 2):22–31; 1992.

Matthew N. Indomethacin responsive headache syndrome. Headache. 21:147–150; 1981.

Mathew NT, Hurt W. Percutaneous radiofrequency trigeminal gangliorhizolysis in intractable cluster headache. Headache. 28:328–331; 1988.

Meyer JS, Hardenberg J. Clinical effectiveness of calcium entry blockers in prophylactic treatment of migraine and cluster headaches. Headache. 23:266–277; 1983.

Meyer JS, Nance M, Walker M, Zetusky WJ, Dowell Jr RE. Migraine and cluster headache treatment with calcium antagonists supports a vascular pathogenesis. Headache. 25:358–367; 1985.

Mullally WJ, Livingstone KR. The treatment of chronic cluster headache with nifedipine. Headache. 24:264–265; 1984.

Onofrio BM, Campbell JK. Surgical treatment of chronic cluster headache. Mayo Clin Proc. 61:537–544; 1986.

Raskin NH. Cluster headache. In: Headache. New York; Churchill Livingstone: 243–244; 1988.

Saper J. Cluster headache. In: Headache Disorders. Boston; John Wright: 108–109; 1983.

Solomon S, Karfunkel P, Guglielmo JM. Migraine-cluster headache syndrome. Headache. 25:236–239; 1985.

Stagliano R, Gallagher RM. Combination ergotamine and lithium therapy in the chronic cluster headache patient. Headache. 23:147; 1983.

Sumatriptan Cluster Headache Study Group. Treatment of acute cluster headache with sumatriptan. N Engl J Med. 6:322–326; 1991.

Wilkins RH, Morgenlander JC. Results of surgical treatment of cluster headache: initial relief followed by recurrence. Neurosurgery. 24:948–951; 1989.

Headache in Children and Adolescents

Allen KD, McKeen LR. Home-based multicomponent treatment of pediatric migraine. Headache. 31:467–472; 1991.

Andrasik F, Kabela E, Quinn S, et al. Psychological functioning of children who have recurrent migraine. Pain. 34:43–52; 1988.

Barlow CF. Headaches and Migraine in Children. J.B. Lippincott; Philadelphia: 1984.

Bille B, Ludbigsson J, Sannerg G. Prophylaxis of migraine in children. Headache. 17:61–63; 1977.

Carter CM, Egger J, Soothill JF. A dietary management of severe childhood migraine. Human Nutrit Appl Nutrit. 39A:294–303; 1985.

Chu ML, Shinnar S. Headaches in children younger than 7 years of age. Headache Quarterly, Cur Tx & Res. 3(2):223; 1992.

Cunningham SJ, McGrath PJ, Ferguston HB, et al. Personality and behavioural characteristics in pediatric migraine. Headache. 27:16–20, 1987.

Engel JM, Rapoff MA, Pressman AR. Long-term follow-up of relaxation training for pediatric headache disorders. Headache. 32:152–156; 1992.

Elser JM, Woody RC. Migraine headache in the infant and young child. Headache. 30:366–368; 1990.

Forsythe WI, Gillies D, Sills MA. Propranolol (Inderal) in the treatment of childhood migraine. Dev Med Child Neurol. 26:737–741; 1984.

Gascon GG. Chronic and recurrent headaches in children and adolescents. Pediatr Clin North Am. 31:1027–1051; 1984.

Hockaday JM. Migraine in Childhood. Butterworth; London: 1988.

Jay GW, Tomasi LG. Pediatric headaches: a one-year retrospective analysis. Headache. 21:5–9; 1981.

Larsson B, Melin L, Deberl A. Recurrent tension headache in adolescents treated with self-help relaxation training and a muscle relaxant drug. Headache. 30:665–671; 1990.

Marcon RA, Labbo EE. Assessment and treatment of children's headaches from a developmental perspective. Headache. 30:586–592; 1990.

Olness KN, McDonald JT. Return headaches in children—diagnosis and treatment. Peds Rev. 8:307–311; 1987.

Prensky AL. Migraine and migrainous variants in pediatric patients. Ped Clin N Am. 23(3):461–471; 1976.

Prensky AL, Sommer D. Diagnosis and treatment of migraine in children. Neurology. 29:506–510; 1979.

Rothner AD. Diagnosis and Management of Headache in Children and Adolescents, Neurologic Clinics. Philadelphia; W.B. Saunders: 1:511–526; 1983.

Rothner AD. The migraine syndrome in children and adolescents. Ped Neurology. 2:3.

Rothner AD. Comparing Childhood and Adult Migraine, Syllabus. American Academy of Neurologists 40th Annual Meeting, Cincinnati, Ohio, April 1988.

Silberstein SD. Twenty questions about headaches in children and adolescents. Headache. 30:716–724; 1990.

Sillanpoo P, Piekkala P, Kero P. Prevalence of headache at preschool age in an unselected child population. Headache Quarterly, Cur Tx & Res. 3(2):223; 1992.

Sillanpoo M, Piekkala P, Kero P. Prevalence of headache at preschool age in an unselected child population. Cephalalgia. 11:239–242; 1991.

Miscellaneous Headache Topics

Abouleish E, de la Vega S, Blendinger I, Tio T. Long-term follow-up of epidural blood patch. Anesth Analg. 54:459–463; 1975.

Anthony M. Arrest of attacks of cluster headache by local steroid injection of the occipital nerve. In: Migraine: Clinical and Research Advances. FC Rose, ed. Basel; Karger: 169–173; 1985.

Bart AJ, Wheeler AS. Comparison of epidural saline placement and epidural blood placement in the treatment of post lumbar puncture headache. Anesthesiology. 48:221–223; 1978.

Bartleson JD. Transient and persistent neurologic manisfestations of migraine. Curr Concepts Cerebrovasc Dis Stroke. 15:383–386; 1984.

Baysinger CL, Menk EJ, Harte E, Middaugh R. The successful treatment of dural puncture headache after failed epidural blood patch. Anesth Analg. 65:1242–1244; 1986.

Bennett DR, Fuenning SI, Sullivan G, Weber J. Migraine precipitated by head trauma in athletes. Am J Sports Med. 8:202–205; 1980.

Blau JN, Engel H. Episodic paroxysmal hemicrania: a further case and review of the literature. Headache Quarterly, Cur Tx & Res. 2(1):61; 1991.

Bogduk N. The anatomy of occipital neuralgia. Clin Exp Neuro. 17:167–184; 1980.

Boghen D, Desauliners N. Background vascular headache: relief with indomethacin. Can J Neurol Sci. 10:270–271; 1983.

Bovim G, Fredriksen TA, Stolt-Nielsen A, Sjaastad O. Neuroloysis of the greater occipital nerve in cervicogenic headache. A follow-up study. Headache. 32:175–179; 1992.

Braun A, Klawans HL. Headaches associated with exercise and sexual activity. In: Handbook of Clinical Neurology, Vol. 38. FC Rose, ed. Amsterdam; Elsevier Science Publishers: 373–382; 1986.

Cornwall RD, Dolan WM. Radicular back pain following lumbar epidural blood patch. Anesthesiology. 43:692–693; 1975.

Crawford JS. Experiences with epidural blood patch. Anesthesia. 35:513–515; 1980.

Di Giovani AJ, Galbert MW, Wahle WM. Epidural injection of autologous blood for postlumbar-puncture headache. Anesth Analg. 51:226–232; 1972.

Diamond S. Prolonged benign exertional headache: its clinical characteristics and response to indomethacin. Headache. 22:96–98; 1982.

Diamond S, Medina JL. Benign exertional headache: successful treatment with indomethacin. Headache. 19:249; 1979.

Dugan MD, Locke S, Gallagher JR. Occipital neuralgia in adolescents and young adults. N Engl J Med. 267:1166–1172; 1962.

Easton JD. Headache after lumbar puncture. Lancet. 1:974–975; 1979.

Edmeads J. Headache and head pains associated with diseases of the cervical spine. Med Clin North Am. 62:533–544; 1978.

Edmeads J. The headaches of ischemic cerebrovascular disease. Headache. 19:345–349; 1979.

Fleetcroft R, Maddocks JL. Headache due to ischemic heart disease. J R Soc Med. 76:676; 1985.

Gaukroger PB, Brownridge P. Epidural blood patch in the treatment of spontaneous low CSF pressure headache. Pain. 29:119–122; 1987.

Gawel MJ, Rothbart PJ. Occipital nerve block in the management of headache and cervical pain. Headache Quarterly, Cur Tx & Res. 3(3):349; 1992.

Haas DC, Pineda GS, Lourie H. Juvenile head trauma syndromes and their relationship to migraine. Arch Neurol. 32:727–730; 1975.

Hale WE, May FE, Marks RG, Moore MT, Stewart RB. Headache in the elderly: an evaluation of risk factors. Headache. 27:272–276; 1987.

Hammond SR, Danta G. Occipital neuralgia. Clin Exp Neurol. 15:258–270; 1978.

Hannerz J, Ericson K, Bergstrand G. Chronic paroxysmal hemicrania: orbital pflebography and steriod treatment. Cephalalgia. 7:189–192; 1987.

Hilton-Jones D. What is postlumbar puncture headache and is it avoidable? In: Dilemmas in the Management of the Neurological Patient. C Warlow, J Garfield, eds. New York; Churchill Livingstone: 144–157; 1984.

Jacome DE. Basilar artery migraine after uncomplicated whiplash injuries. Headache. 26:515–516; 1986.

Jensen NB, Joensen P, Jensen J. Chronic paroxysmal hemicrania: continued remission of symptoms after discontinuation of indomethacin. Cephalalgia. 2:163–164; 1982.

Jotkowitz S. Chronic paroxysmal hemicrania and cluster. Ann Neurol. 4:389; 1978.

Kelly R. The post-traumatic syndrome. Proc R Soc Med. 24:242–244; 1981.

Khurana RK. Post-traumatic headache with ptosis, miosis and chronic forehead hyperhidrosis. Headache. 30:64–68; 1990.

Kuritzky A. Indomethacin-resistant hemicrania continua. Headache Quarterly, Cur Tx & Res. 3(3):351; 1992.

Lance JW. Headaches related to sexual activity. J Neurol Neurosurg Psych. 39:1226–1230; 1976.

Loeb C, Gandolfo C, Dall'Agata D. Headache in transient ischemic attack (TIA). Cephalagia. 2(Suppl):17–19; 1985.

Mathew NT. Indomethacin responsive headache syndromes. Headache. 21:147–150; 1981.

McKinlay WW, Brooks DN, Bond MR. Postconcussional symptoms, financial compensation and outcome of severe blunt head injury. J Neurol Neurosurg Psych. 46:1084–1091; 1983.

Medina JL. Organic headaches mimicking chronic paroxysmal hemicrania. Headache Quarterly, Cur Tx & Res. 3(3):351; 1992.

Medina JL, Diamond S. Cluster headache variant: spectrum of a new headache syndrome. Arch Neurol. 38:708–709; 1981.

Medina J, Diamond S, Rubino F. Headache in patients with transient ischemic attacks. Headache. 15:194–197; 1975.

Newman LC, Lipton RB, Russell M, Solomon S. Hemicrania continua: attacks may alternate sides. Headache. 32:237–238; 1992.

Olsen KS. Epidural blood patch in the treatment of post-lumbar puncture headache. Pain. 30:293–301; 1987.

Parris WCV. Use of the epidural blood patch in the treatment of chronic headaches. Anesthesiology. 65:344; 1986.

Paulson GW, Klawans HL. Benign orgasmic cephalgia. Headache. 13:181–187; 1974.

Portendy RK, Abissi CJ, Lipton RB, et al. Headache in cerebrovascular disease. Stroke. 15:1009–1012; 1984.

Raskin NH. Repetitive intravenous dihydroergotamine as treatment for intractable migraine. Neurology. 36:995–997; 1986.

Rooke ED. Benign exertional headache. Med Clin North Am. 52:801–808; 1968.

Russell D. Chronic paroxysmal hemicrania: severity, duration and time of occurrences of attacks. Cephalalgia. 4:53–56; 1984.

Saadah HA, Taylor FB. Sustained headache syndrome associated with tender occipital nerve zones. Headache. 27:201–205; 1987.

Sechzer PG, Abel L. Post-spinal anesthesia headache treated with caffeine. Evaluation with demand method, part 1. Curr Ther Res. 24:307–312; 1978.

Serratrice G, Serbanesco F, Sambuc R. Epidemiology of headache in elderly— correlations with life conditions and socio-professional environment. Headache. 25:85–89; 1985.

Sjaastad O. Chronic paroxysmal hemicrania. In: Handbook of Clinical Neurology, Vol. 48. FC Rose, ed. Amsterdam; Elsevier Science Publishing: 257–266; 1986.

Sjaastad O, Spierings ELH. "Hemicrania continua": another headache absolutely responsive to indomethacin. Cephalalgia. 4:65–70; 1984.

Sjaastad O, Saunte C, Graham JR. Chronic paroxysmal hemicrainia. VII. Mechanical precipitation of attacks: new cases and localization of trigger points. Cephalalgia. 4:113–118; 1984.

Sjaastad O, Antonaci F. Chronic paroxysmal hemicrania. Long-lasting remission in the chronic stage. Cephalalgia. 7:203–205; 1987.

Smith FR, Perkin GD, Rose FC. Posture and headache after lumbar puncture. Lancet. 1:1245; 1980.

Takeshima T, Taniguchi R, Kitagawa T, Takahashi K. Headaches in dementia. Headache. 30:735–738; 1990.

Tarsh MJ, Royston C. A follow-up study of accident neurosis. Br J Psych. 146:18–25; 1985.

Traub YM, Korczyn AD. Headache in patients with hypertension. Headache. 17:245–247; 1978.

Tyler GS, McNeely HE, Dick ML. Treatment of post-traumatic headache with amitripyline. Headache. 20:213–216; 1980.

Vijayan N, Dreyfus PM. Post-traumatic dysautonomic cephalgia. Arch Neurol. 32:649–652; 1975.

Weiss HD, Stern BJ, Goldberg J. Post-traumatic migraine: chronic migraine precipitated by minor head or neck trauma. Headache. 31:451–456; 1991.

Drug Identification Guide and Index

For Medications Used by Headache Patients

Adapin Capsules
  10 mg, gold
  25 mg, lime and gold
  50 mg, lime
  75 mg, gold and white
  100 mg, lime and white
  150 mg, tan and cream
Adapin Tablets
  25 mg, white, oval, scored
Advil Caplets
  200 mg, brown, oval
Advil Liquid
  100 mg/5 cc
Advil Tablets
  200 mg, brown, round
Anacin Caplets
  white, capsule-shaped
Anacin Capsules
  yellow and white
Anacin Maximum Strength Tablets
  white, round
Anacin-3 Maximum Strength Caplets
  500 mg, white, capsule-shaped
Anacin-3 Maximum Strength Tablets
  500 mg, white, round
Anaprox Tablets
  275 mg, light blue, oval
Anaprox DS Tablets
  550 mg, dark blue, capsule-shaped
Ansaid Tablets
  50 mg, white oval
  100 mg, blue oval

Asendin Tablets
  25 mg, white, heptagonal, scored
  50 mg, orange, heptagonal, scored
  100 mg, blue, heptagonal, scored
  150 mg, peach, heptagonal, scored
Ativan Tablets
  0.5 mg, white, five-sided
  1 mg, white, five-sided, scored
  2 mg, white, five-sided, scored
Aventyl HCI Pulvules
  10 mg, yellow and white
  25 mg, yellow and white
Axotal Tablets
  white, capsule-shaped
Bayer Aspirin Tablets, Maximum
  500 mg, white, round
Bayer Timed-Release Aspirin Tablets, 8-Hour
  650 mg, white, oblong, scored
Bellergal-S Tablets
  dark green, orange, light lemon yellow, mottled, round, scored
Blocadren Tablets
  5 mg, light blue, round
  10 mg, light blue, round, scored
  20 mg, light blue, capsule-shaped, scored
Bufferin Arthritis Strength Caplets
  white, capsule-shaped
Bufferin Extra-Strength Tablets
  white, capsule-shaped
Bufferin Tablets
  white, round
BuSpar Tablets
  5 mg, white, ovoid-rectangular, scored
  10 mg, white, ovoid-rectangular, scored
Cafergot Suppositories
Cafergot PB Suppositories (only generic available, or through compounding phar-
    macists)
Cafergot Tablets
  shell pink, round
Calan Tablets
  40 mg, pink, round
  80 mg, peach, oval, scored
  120 mg, brown, oval, scored
Calan SR Caplets
  120 mg
  180 mg, light pink, oval, scored
  240 mg, light green capsule-shaped, scored
Cardizem Tablets
  30 mg, green, round
  60 mg, yellow, round, scored

90 mg, green, oblong, scored
120 mg, yellow, oblong, scored
Cardizem SR Capsules
    60 mg, brown and ivory
    90 mg, brown and gold
    120 mg, brown and caramel
Compazine Spansules
    10 mg, black and clear with light green beads
    15 mg, black and clear with light green beads
    30 mg, black and clear with light green beads
Compazine Suppositories
    25 mg
Compazine Tablets
    5 mg, yellow-green, round
    10 mg, yellow-green, round
    25 mg, yellow-green, round
Corgard Tablets
    20 mg, sky blue, round, scored
    40 mg, sky blue, round, scored
    80 mg, light blue, round, scored
    120 mg, powder blue, capsule-shaped, scored
    160 mg, sky blue, capsule-shaped, scored
Dalmane Capsules
    15 mg, orange and ivory
    30 mg, red and ivory
Danocrine Capsules
    50 mg, orange and white
    100 mg, yellow
    200 mg, orange
Darvocet-N 100 Tablets
    orange, oblong
Darvon Pulvules
    65 mg, light pink
Darvon Compound Pulvules
    light grey and light pink
Darvon Compound-65 Pulvules
    light grey and red
Darvon-N Tablets
    100 mg, buff, oval
Decadron Tablets
    0.25 mg, orange, pentagonal, scored
    0.5 mg, yellow, pentagonal, scored
    0.75 mg, bluish-green, pentagonal, scored
    1.5 mg, pink, pentagonal, scored
    4 mg, white, pentagonal, scored
    6 mg, green, pentagonal, scored
Deltasone Tablets
    2.5 mg, pink, round, scored
    5 mg, white, round, scored

10 mg, white, round, scored
20 mg, peach, round, scored
50 mg, white, round, scored
Demerol Tablets
   50 mg, white, round, scored
   100 mg, white, round
Depakene Capsules
   250 mg, orange
Depakote Sprinkle Capsules
   125 mg, opaque white and blue
Depakote Tablets
   125 mg, salmon pink, oval
   250 mg, peach, oval
   500 mg, lavender, oval
Desyrel Dividose Tablets
   150 mg, orange, oblong, triple-scored
   300 mg, yellow, oblong, triple-scored
Desyrel Tablets
   50 mg, peach, round, scored
   100 mg, white, round, scored
Diamox Sequels
   500 mg, orange
Diamox Tablets
   125 mg, white, round, scored
   250 mg, white, round, double-scored
Dilaudid Tablets
   1 mg, green, round
   2 mg, orange, round
   3 mg, pink, round
   4 mg, yellow, round
Disalcid Capsules
   500 mg, aqua and white
Disalcid Tablets
   500 mg, light blue, round
   750 mg, light blue, capsule-shaped, scored
Dolobid Tablets
   250 mg, peach, capsule-shaped
   500 mg, orange, capsule-shaped
Ecotrin Caplets
   325 mg, orange, capsule-shaped
   500 mg, orange, capsule-shaped
Ecotrin Tablets
   325 mg, orange, round
   500 mg, orange, round
Elavil Tablets
   10 mg, blue, round
   25 mg, yellow, round
   50 mg, beige, round
   75 mg, orange, round

100 mg, mauve, round

150 mg, blue, capsule-shaped

Empirin with Codeine No. 2 Tablets

white, round

Empirin with Codeine No. 3 Tablets

white, round

Empirin with Codeine No. 4 Tablets

white, round

Endep Tablets

10 mg, orange, round, scored

25 mg, orange, round, scored

50 mg, orange, round, scored

75 mg, yellow, round, scored

100 mg, peach, round, scored

150 mg, salmon, round, scored

Equagesic Tablets

yellow and pink, layered, round, scored

Ergonovine Capsules

0.2 mg, (formulated by compounding pharmacists)

Ergostat Sublingual Tablets

2 mg, orange, round

Esgic Capsules

white

Esgic Tablets

white, round Esgic Plus-White, oblong

Eskalith Capsules

300 mg, grey and yellow

Eskalith Tablets

300 mg, grey, round, scored

Eskalith CR Tablets

450 mg, buff, round, scored

Estinyl Tablets

0.02 mg, beige, round

0.05 mg, pink, round

0.5 mg, peach, round, scored

Estrace Tablets

1 mg, lavender, round, scored

2 mg, turquoise, round, scored

Estraderm Transdemal Systems

0.05 mg/24 hour

0.1 mg/24 hour

Estratab tablets

0.625 mg, yellow, round

1.25 mg, red-orange, round

2.5 mg, sugar pink, round

Estratest Tablets

dark green, oval

Estratest H.S. Tablets

light green, oval

Excedrin, Aspirin Free
Excedrin, Extra-Strength
Excedrin P.M. Aspirin Free Caplets
  blue, capsule-shaped
Fioricet Tablets
  light blue, round
Fiorinal Capsules
  bright Kelly green and lime green
Fiorinal Tablets
  white, round
Fiorinal with Codeine No. 3 Capsules
  blue and yellow
Flexeril Tablets
  10 mg, butterscotch yellow, D-shaped
Halcion Tablets
  0.125 mg, pale lavender, oval
  0.25 mg, powder blue, oval, scored
Hydrocet Capsules
  blue and white
Inderal Tablets
  10 mg, orange, hexagonal, scored
  20 mg, blue, hexagonal, scored
  40 mg, green, hexagonal, scored
  60 mg, pink, hexagonal, scored
  80 mg, yellow, hexagonal, scored
Inderal LA Capsules
  60 mg, white and blue with white and blue bands
  80 mg, right blue
  120 mg, dark blue and light blue
  160 mg, dark blue
Indocin Capsules
  25 mg, blue and white
  50 mg, blue and white
Indocin SR Capsules
  75 mg, blue and clear with blue and white beads
Isoptin Tablets
  40 mg, blue, round, scored
  80 mg, yellow, round, scored
  120 mg, white, round, scored
Isoptin SR Tablets
  120 mg, light pink, capsule-shaped
  180 mg, light pink, capsule-shaped, scored
  240 mg, yellow, capsule-shaped, scored
Klonopin Tablets
  0.5 mg, orange, round, scored
  1 mg, blue, round, scored
  2 mg, white, round, scored
Librium Capsules
  5 mg, green and yellow

10 mg, black and green
25 mg, green and white
Limbitrol Tablets
  blue, round
Limbitrol D.S. Tablets
  white, round
Lithobid SR Tablets
  300 mg, peach, round
Lithonate Capsules
  300 mg, peach
Lithotabs Tablets
  300 mg, white, round, scored
Lopressor Tablets
  50 mg, light red, capsule-shaped, scored
  100 mg, light blue, capsule-shaped, scored
Marplan Tablets
  10 mg, peach, round, scored
Meclomen Capsules
  50 mg, orange and light orange
  100 mg, orange and beige
Medipren Caplets
  200 mg, white, capsule-shaped, scored
Medipren Tablets
  200 mg, white, round
Medrol Tablets
  2 mg, pink, oval, scored
  4 mg, white, oval, scored
  8 mg, peach, oval, scored
  16 mg, white, oval, scored
  24 mg, light yellow, oval, scored
  32 mg, peach, oval, scored
Mepergan Fortis Capsules
  maroon
Methergine Tablets
  0.2 mg, rose, round
Midol Caplets
  white, capsule-shaped
Midol Maximum Strength Tablets
  white, capsule-shaped
Midrin Capsules
  red with pink band
Miltown Tablets
  200 mg, white, round
  400 mg, white, round
Moduretic Tablets
  peach, diamond-shaped
Motrin Tablets
  300 mg, white, round
  400 mg, orange, round

600 mg, peach, oval
800 mg, apricot, capsule-shaped
Motrin IB Caplets
200 mg, white, capsule-shaped
Motrin IB Tablets
200 mg, white, round
Nalfon Pulvules
300 mg, ocher and yellow
Nalfon Tablets
600 mg, yellow, capsule-shaped, scored
Nalfon 200 Pulvules
200 mg, ocher and white
Naprosyn Tablets
250 mg, yellow, round, scored
375 mg, peach, oval
500 mg, yellow, oval
Nardil Tablets
15 mg, orange, round
Nolvadex Tablets
10 mg, white, round, cameo-debossed
Norflex Tablets
100 mg, white, round
Norgesic Tablets
light green, white, and yellow, layered, round
Norgesic Forte Tablets
light green, white, and yellow, layered, capsule-shaped, scored
Norpramin Tablets
10 mg, blue, round
25 mg, yellow, round
50 mg, green, round
75 mg, red, round
100 mg, peach, round
150 mg, white, round
Nuprin Tablets
200 mg, yellow, round
Orudis Capsules
25 mg, green and red
50 mg, dark green and light green
75 mg, dark green and white
Pamelor Capsules
10 mg, orange and white
25 mg, orange and white
50 mg, white
75 mg, orange and white
Panadol Junior Strength Caplets
160 mg, white, capsule-shaped, scored
Parafon Forte DSC Caplets
500 mg, light green, capsule-shaped, scored
Pepcid Tablets

20 mg, beige, U-shaped
40 mg, light brownish orange, U-shaped
Percocet Tablets
  white, round, scored
Percodan Tablets
  yellow, round, scored
Percodan-Demi Tablets
  pink, round, scored
Percogesic Tablets
  light orange, mottled, round, scored
Periactin Tablets
  4 mg, white, round, scored
Phenaphen 650 with Codeine Tablets
  white, capsule-shaped, scored
Phenaphen with Codeine No. 2 Capsules
  black and yellow
Phenaphen with Codeine No. 3 Capsules
  black and green
Phenaphen with Codeine No. 4 Capsules
  green and white
Phenergan Suppositories
  25 mg
  50 mg
Phenergan Tablets
  12.5 mg, orange, round, scored
  25 mg, white, round, quarter-scored
  50 mg, pink, round
Phenergan-D Tablets
  white and orange, layered, round, scored
Phrenilin Tablets
  pale violet, round, scored
Phrenilin Forte Capsules
  amethyst
Ponstel Kapseals
  250 mg, yellow with blue band
Premarin Tablets
  0.3 mg, green, oval
  0.625 mg, maroon, oval
  0.9 mg, white, oval
  1.25 mg, yellow, oval
  2.5 mg, purple, oval
Procardia Capsules
  10 mg, orange
  20 mg, two-tone orange, oval
Procardia XL Tablets
  30 mg, rose-pink, round
  60 mg, rose-pink, round
  90 mg, rose-pink, round

Prozac Capsules
   10 to 20 mg, green and off-white
Prozac Liquid
   10 mg/5 cc
Quinamm Tablets
   260 mg, round, white
Reglan Tablets
   5 mg, green, elliptical-shaped
   10 mg, white, capsule-shaped, scored
Rufen Tablets
   400 mg, pink, round
   600 mg, white, oblong
   800 mg, white, oblong
Sansert Tablets
   2 mg, yellow, round
Serax Capsules
   10 mg, pink and white
   15 mg, red and white
   30 mg, maroon and white
Sinarest Extra-Strength Tablets
   yellow, oval
Sinarest Sinus Relief Tablets
   yellow, round
Sine-Off Extra Strength, No Drowsiness Aspirin-Free Capsules
   red
Sine-Off Regular Strength with Aspirin Tablets
   yellow, round
Sinequan Capsules
   10 mg, red and pink
   25 mg, blue and pink
   50 mg, pink and light pink
   75 mg, light pink
   100 mg, blue and light pink
   150 mg, blue
Sinubid Tablets
   pink and light pink, layered, ellipsoid, scored
Sinulin Tablets
   peach, round, scored
Sinutab Allergy Formula Tablets
   green, round
Sinutab Maximum Strength Tablets
   yellow, oval
Sinutab Maximum Strength Without Drowsiness Tablets
   peach, oval
Sinutab Without Drowsiness Tablets
   pink, round, scored
Skelaxin Tablets
   400 mg, pale rose, round, scored

Soma Tablets
  350 mg, white, round
Soma Compound Tablets
  white and orange, layered, round
Sparine Tablets
  25 mg, yellow, round
  50 mg, orange, round
  100 mg, pink, round
Sudafed Tablets
  30 mg, red, round
  60 mg, white, round
Sudafed 12-Hour Capsules
  red and clear with white beads and blue band
Sudafed Plus Tablets
  white, round, scored
Sudafed Sinus Caplets
  peach, mottled, capsule-shaped
Sudafed Sinus Tablets
  peach, mottled, round
Surmontil Capsules
  25 mg, blue and yellow
  50 mg, blue and orange
  100 mg, blue and white
Synalgos-DC Capsules
  blue and gray
Synthroid Tablets
  25 micrograms, orange, round, scored
  50 micrograms, white, round, scored
  75 micrograms, violet, round, scored
  88 micrograms, olive, round, scored
  100 micrograms, yellow, round, scored
  125 micrograms, brown, round, scored
  150 micrograms, blue, round, scored
  200 micrograms, pink, round, scored
  300 micrograms, green, round, scored
Tagamet Tablets
  200 mg, pale green, round
  300 mg, pale green, round
  400 mg, pale green, oblong
  800 mg, pale green, oval, scored
Talacen Caplets
  pale blue, capsule-shaped, scored
Talwin Nx Tablets
  yellow, oblong, scored
Tegretol Chewable Tablets
  100 mg, white with pink mottling, scored
Tegretol Tablets
  200 mg, pink, capsule-shaped, scored

Tenormin Tablets
  25 mg, white, round, scored
  50 mg, white, round, scored
  100 mg, white, round
Thorazine Spansules
  30 mg, orange and clear with pale pink and white beads
  75 mg, orange and clear with pale pink and white beads
  150 mg, orange and clear with pale pink and white beads
  200 mg, orange and clear with pale pink and white beads
  300 mg, orange and clear with pale pink and white beads
Thorazine Suppositories
  25 mg
  100 mg
Thorazine Tablets
  10 mg, orange, round
  25 mg, orange, round
  50 mg, orange, round
  100 mg, brown, round
  200 mg, orange, round
Tigan Capsules
  100 mg, blue and white
  250 mg, blue
Tigan Suppositories
  100 mg
  250 mg
Tofranil Tablets
  10 mg, coral, triangular
  25 mg, coral, round
  50 mg, coral, round
Tofranil-PM Capsules
  75 mg, coral
  100 mg, coral and dark yellow
  125 mg, coral and light yellow
  150 mg, coral
Tolectin Tablets
  200 mg, white, round, scored
  600 mg, orange, oval
Tolectin DS Capsules
  400 mg, orange with purple-gray parallel bands
Tranxene-SD Tablets
  11.25 mg, blue, round
  22.5 mg, tan, round
Tranxene T-Tab Tablets
  3.75 mg, blue, T-shaped, scored
  7.5 mg, peach, T-shaped, scored
  15 mg, lavender, T-shaped, scored
Triavil 2–10 Tablets
  blue, triangular

Triavil 2–25 Tablets
    orange, triangular
Triavil 4–10 Tablets
    salmon, triangular
Triavil 4–25 Tablets
    yellow, triangular
Triavil 4–50 Tablets
    orange, diamond-shaped
Trilafon Tablets
    2 mg, grey, round
    4 mg, grey, round
    8 mg, grey, round
    16 mg, grey, round
Trilisate 500 Tablets
    500 mg, pale pink, capsule-shaped, scored
Trilisate 750 Tablets
    750 mg, white, capsule-shaped, scored
Trilisate 1,000 Tablets
    1,000 mg, red, capsule-shaped, scored
Tums Tablets
    500 mg, white, round
Tylenol Children's Chewable Tablets
    80 mg, pink, mottled, round, scored
Tylenol Extra Strength Caplets
    500 mg, white, capsule-shaped
Tylenol Extra Strength Tablets
    500 mg, white, round
Tylenol Gelcaps
    500 mg, red and yellow
Tylenol Junior Strength Caplets
    160 mg, white, capsule-shaped, scored
Tylenol Regular Strength Caplets
    325 mg, white, capsule-shaped, scored
Tylenol Regular Strength Tablets
    325 mg, white, round, scored
Tylenol Allergy Sinus Caplets
    yellow, capsule-shaped
Tylenol Children's Cold Chewable Tablets
    purple, round
Tylenol Cold Multi-Symptom Tablets
    yellow, round
Tylenol Cold No Drowsiness Formula Caplets
    white, capsule-shaped
Tylenol with Codeine No. 3 Capsules
    white with red bands
Tylenol with Codeine No. 4 Capsules
    red
Tylenol with Codeine No. 1 Tablets
    white, round

Tylenol with Codeine No. 2 Tablets
  white, round
Tylenol with Codeine No. 3 Tablets
  white, round
Tylenol with Codeine No. 4 Tablets
  white, round
Tylox Capsules
  red
Valium Tablets
  2 mg, white, round with V-shaped cutout, scored
  5 mg, Yellow, round with V-shaped cutout, scored
  10 mg, blue, round with V-shaped cutout, scored
Valrelease Capsules
  15 mg, blue and yellow
Vicodin Tablets
  white, capsule-shaped, scored
Vicodin ES
  white, oval, bevelled, scored
Vistaril Capsules
  25 mg, dark green and light green
  50 mg, green and white
  100 mg, gray and green
Vivactil Tablets
  5 mg, orange, oval
  10 mg, yellow, oval
Voltaren Tablets
  25 mg, yellow, round
  50 mg, light brown, round
  75 mg, white, round
Wellbutrin Tablets
  75 mg, yellow-gold, round
  100 mg, red, round
Wigraine Rectal Suppositories
  white, oval
Wigraine Tablets
  white, round
Xanax Tablets
  0.25 mg, white, oval, scored
  0.5 mg, peach, oval, scored
  1 mg, lavender, oval, scored
  2 mg, white, oblong, scored
Zantac 150 Tablets
  150 mg, white, round
Zantac 300 Tablets
  300 mg, yellow, capsule-shaped
Zoloft 50 and 100 mg tablets, scored

Headache Calendar for Patients

At times, charting the headaches and trigger factors may help the patient and physician. The headache calendar is particularly useful in new onset headaches. The following is a sample headache calendar for patients.

Name_____ HEADACHE CALENDAR

Headache Trigger Factors: (1) Stress, (2) After stress is over, (3) Foods, such as chocolate or wine, (4) Weather changes, (5) Missing a meal, (6) (in women) Menstrual or premenstrual days, or hormone changes, such as with the birth control pill or during menopause, (7) Bright lights or sunlight, (8) Perfumes or other odors, (9) Undersleeping, (10) Oversleeping, (11) Exercise or exertion, (12) Cigarette smoke, (13) Traveling, such as flying or car rides.

Overall Severity of the Headache That Day
Severity Scale

1	5	10
none	mild	moderate	severe

In the "overall severity #" column below, put one number down for how the whole day was, overall.

Date	Trigger Factor#	Overall Severity#	"As Needed" Medicine, & Did It Help

Foods to Avoid
(For Migraine Patients)

In many migraineurs, dietary trigger factors will occasionally bring on a headache. The degree of sensitivity to foods varies widely among migraine sufferers. The mechanism of food-provoked headaches is probably not an allergy, but rather a sensitivity to chemicals in the foods, such as tyramine, phenylethylamine (in chocolate), and monosodium glutamate. Nitrites may also be a problem.

The headache will usually begin soon after ingestion of the offending substance, but there may be a delay of hours. At certain times, patients may be more susceptible to the foods, such as a female migraineur around menstruation.

The following is a list of foods that, at times, may trigger headaches.

Foods to Avoid

Foods that are Extremely Common Migraine Triggers (The Worst Offenders)

Monosodium Glutamate (MSG): also labeled Autolyzed Yeast Extract, Hydrolyzed Vegetable Protein or Natural Flavoring. Possible sources of MSG include: broths or stocks, seasonings, whey protein, soy extract, malt extract, caseinate, barley extract, textured soy protein, chicken or pork or beef flavoring, smoke flavor, spices, carrageenan, meat tenderizer, seasoned salt, TV dinners, instant gravies, and some potato chips and dry-roasted nuts.

Red wine

Beer

Chocolate

Citrus fruits

Ripened, aged cheeses (Colby, Roquefort, brie, Gruyere, cheddar, bleu, brick, mozzarella, Parmesan, boursalt, Romano), and processed cheese Less likely to trigger headache: Cottage cheese, cream cheese, and American cheese

Hot dogs, pepperoni, bologna, salami, sausage, canned or cured meats (bacon, ham), aged meats, or marinated meats

Foods that Trigger Migraines Less Often
(Moderate Offenders)

White wine
Alcohol (miscellaneous); vodka is the least likely to bring on migraine
Cocoa
Buttermilk
Fresh, hot homemade yeast breads (once cooled they are OK)
Sour cream
Yogurt
Soy sauce
Caffeine: caffeine often helps headaches, and is contained in many migraine
  medications. However, some people cannot tolerate even small amounts of
  caffeine; overuse of caffeine also leads to rebound (increased) headaches
Yeast extracts
Acidophilus milk
Peanuts, Peanut Butter
Nuts or seeds (any may trigger migraine)

Foods that Occasionally Trigger Migraines
(Mild Offenders)

Onions
Certain beans: lima, navy, lentils, Italian, fava, garbanzo, pinto, and snow peas
Sauerkraut
Pickles
Chile peppers
Licorice or carob candy
Liver
Figs
Fried foods
Popcorn
Sugar in excess
Salt in excess
Seafood
Pork
Aspartame

Relaxation Exercises for Headache Patients

Headache sufferers need to be offered relaxation exercises as an adjunct to medicine, particularly for stressful situations and tension headaches. We do not want patients reaching for the analgesics all day. If they are offered simple exercises that may be performed in 20 or 30 seconds, the relaxation may help to decrease the muscular tension about the head, and decrease the headache pain.

In my experience, the overwhelming majority of patients will not follow through with formal biofeedback programs, either because of lack of motivation, time, or money. We need to make available simple techniques that they may learn at home, with minimal therapist assistance.

Relaxation exercises can help with headaches and neck pain, or for general nervousness/anxiety. Some people practice the exercises, particularly deep breathing, for a few minutes each day, whereas others use the exercises for several minutes only when they have a headache. Patients should be encouraged to do 20 or 30 seconds of deep breathing for mild, daily headaches, instead of reaching for an analgesic.

Books or cassette tapes obtained in bookstores are helpful in learning about relaxation. The success of relaxation therapy is directly related to the motivation of the person performing the exercises. If patients will not follow through and regularly practice the exercises, it is pointless for them to waste time with relaxation or biofeedback.

Relaxation exercises are helpful because they relax the muscles around the head and neck, and there may be beneficial vascular effects as well. One or two sessions with a psychotherapist trained in teaching relaxation is very helpful; some patients need multiple sessions in a more formal biofeedback training program.

The following are simple relaxation exercises designed for patients to learn, by themselves, at home.

Deep Breathing

Deep breathing is easy and effective. It can be very helpful for combating stress on a daily basis. Twenty or thirty seconds, or 5 breaths, may be all that is necessary. Patients should be taught to slow their breathing down for $\frac{1}{2}$ minute, focus on the breaths, with eyes closed, and take very deep breaths.

Abdominal breathing may be practiced anywhere, anytime. The easiest position to first learn this technique is lying on the back, as follows:

1. Lie down on your back, with one hand on your abdomen, and one on your chest.
2. Breathe through your nose, slowly.
3. While finishing the breath, push your abdomen with your hand up toward the sky.
4. Slowly allow the breath to pass back out through your chest and nostrils.
5. Do the above daily for as long as you have time (at least several minutes each day).
6. As you exhale, you may find it helpful to say, to yourself, "relax". With practice, 4 or 5 deep breaths, while saying "relax", may be all that is necessary to significantly lower your muscle tension.
7. While inhaling, it may be beneficial to count slowly from 1 to 4, hold the breath for a second, and then exhale, counting from 1 to 7, slowly.

Imagery

Adding imagery to the deep breathing enhances the effectiveness. The following instructions may be given to the patient.

1. Imagine a quiet, calm, pleasant scene. It should be an image that gives you an overall feeling of well-being; examples are a warm, comfortable room with a crackling fire going in the fireplace, lying on a cool, beautiful, spacious expanse of grass, or being on a lovely white sand beach.
2. After beginning the deep breathing, put yourself into the comfortable scene. Attempt to experience all of the sounds, feelings, smells, and intricacies of the image. Continue the deep breathing throughout the entire exercise.

There are many more techniques available, such as progressive muscle relaxation. These techniques are easy to learn, and patients should be encouraged to at least attempt some form of relaxation or biofeedback.

Index